Reader's
Digest Guide to
Eye Care

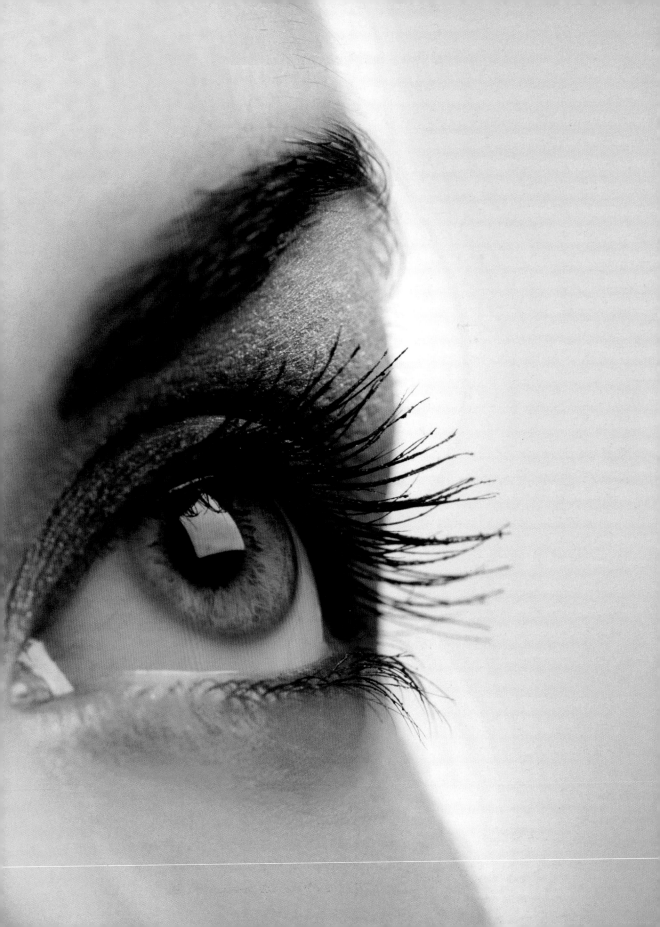

Reader's Digest Guide to Eye Care

Common Vision Problems, from Dry Eye to Macular Degeneration

JENNIFER S. WEIZER, M.D.,
AND JOSHUA D. STEIN, M.D., M.S.

Foreword by Sharon Fekrat, M.D., FACS
Associate Professor of Ophthalmology, Duke Eye Center
Chief, Ophthalmology, Durham Veterans Affairs Medical Center

Reader's Digest

The Reader's Digest Association, Inc.
Pleasantville, New York/Montreal/London/Sydney/Singapore/Mumbai

A READER'S DIGEST BOOK

Copyright © 2009 Quantum Publishing Ltd
This edition published by The Reader's Digest
Association, Inc., by arrangement with
Quantum Publishing Ltd

FOR QUANTUM PUBLISHING
Project Editor Samantha Warrington
Designer Sue Costen
Production Rohana Yusof
Publisher Anastasia Cavouras

FOR READER'S DIGEST
U.S. Project Editor Siobhan Sullivan
Canadian Project Editor Jesse Corbeil
Project Designer Jennifer Tokarski
Senior Art Director George McKeon
Executive Editor, Trade Publishing Dolores York
Associate Publisher Rosanne McManus
President and Publisher, Trade Publishing
Harold Clarke

Library of Congress Cataloging in Publication Data:
Weizer, Jennifer S.
Reader's digest guide to eye care : common vision
problems, from dry eye to macular degeneration /
Jennifer S. Weizer and Joshua D. Stein.
p. cm.
 ISBN 978-1-60652-128-1 (hardcover)
 ISBN 978-1-60652-031-4 (paperback)
1. Eye--Care and hygiene--Popular works. 2. Eye--
Diseases--Popular works.
I. Stein, Joshua D., 1974- II. Title.
RE51.W455 2010
617.7'15--dc22
                    2009027952

We are committed to both the quality of our products
and the service we provide to our customers. We value
your comments, so please feel free to contact us:

The Reader's Digest Association, Inc.
Adult Trade Publishing
Reader's Digest Road
Pleasantville, NY 10570-7000

For more Reader's Digest products and information,
visit our website:

www.rd.com (in the United States)
www.readersdigest.ca (in Canada)
www.readersdigest.co.uk (in the UK)
www.readersdigest.com.au (in Australia)
www.readersdigest.co.nz (in New Zealand)
www.rdasia.com (in Asia)

Printed in Singapore

1 3 5 7 9 10 8 6 4 2 (hardcover)
1 3 5 7 9 10 8 6 4 2 (paperback)

NOTE TO OUR READERS
The information in this book should not be substituted
for, or used to alter, medical therapy without your
doctor's advice. For a specific health problem, consult
your physician for guidance.

Contents

Foreword

When you develop a medical problem of any kind, what you and your family need most is information—trusted, reliable, and complete information. It is important to understand what your condition actually is, how it should be treated, and why it should be treated using one approach instead of another. The more information you can read and digest about your condition, the more in control you will feel and the better off you, your family, and your health care providers will be. Sometimes, however, finding a trusted, reliable, and complete source of such information can be challenging. With the wealth of information available at your fingertips on the Internet, finding the information you need can also be confusing and occasionally misleading.

Reader's Digest Guide to Eye Care is just the resource individuals with eye disease and their family members need. Full of color illustrations and educational figures and diagrams, *Reader's Digest Guide to Eye Care* was written by two accomplished opthalmic specialists and offers trusted and reliable information. The well-organized presentation of the material is colorful and eye-catching. *Reader's Digest Guide to Eye Care* draws you into its pages as soon as you open the book with its captivating style, and it teaches you about the eye and the numerous conditions that can affect it. Peppered with "Test Your Eye Q" questions, this valuable resource allows the reader to remain engaged in the information presented. "Optical Illusion" inserts are present throughout the handy book and dispel common, yet incorrect, beliefs held by many. The editors must be commended for the innovative design used to present a wealth of information in such depth and detail while still keeping the material easy to understand for the reader.

> If you develop an eye disease, learn as much about it as you can and take charge!

It is a book that can and should be read more than once with new information absorbed each time. The first time you read it, you learn the basics. The second time you read it, you absorb the details. The third time you read it, you appreciate the subtleties.

As you navigate the ever-changing health care system as well as the novel medical and surgical treatments being introduced into the medical field, you must be your own advocate. Self-education and developing an understanding of your own medical diagnosis and treatment options empower you to be an effective participant in that care and, in essence, assist the medical team in taking the best care of the particular condition—by taking care of yourself! *Reader's Digest Guide to Eye Care* is a book that belongs in all home libraries and is a must-read, especially for those who are hoping to prevent, or who are challenged by an eye disease.

Sharon Fekrat, M.D., FACS

Associate Professor of Ophthalmology
Duke Eye Center

Chief, Ophthalmology
Durham Veterans Affairs Medical Center

Introduction

In so many ways, the health of your eyes is tied to the health of the rest of your body. Whether it's by eating a balanced diet, not smoking, or faithfully using sun protection, taking care of your general health also benefits the health of your eyes. By focusing your efforts on maximizing your health, your eyes and your body are likely to reward you by functioning at their best, giving you many years of good vision and well-being.

Similarly, because the different parts of your body are inextricably linked, in many instances diseases that affect your general health can involve your eyes, and treating these diseases for the rest of your body can also help you maintain or improve your eyesight. If you have a medical problem that has the potential to threaten your vision, a great first step you can take is to establish a good working relationship with your eye doctor. This leads to coordinated medical care that encourages your eye doctor and your primary care physician to discuss your health with each other, and you and your doctors will benefit from these open channels of communication. This is one of the best things you can do to ensure that you are maximizing your overall health as well as your eye health.

Since our eyes are our windows to the world, we hope this book will guide you in learning more about keeping your eyes healthy and seeing their best.

We've written this book with the goal of illustrating the rich relationship between your eyes and the rest of your body. By exploring ways in which you yourself can keep your eyes healthy over time, we hope to help you take charge of your eye health and so preserve your most important sense of vision. This book is filled with explanations about how your eyes work and what you can do to keep them functioning properly. It also details common eye problems and tells you how to avoid them or to lessen their impact. We've included a section on living with visual impairment, as many people do live with vision that is less than perfect. We've included many practical tips and checklists that make your eye health easy to understand, and we've discussed ways to keep your eyes looking their youthful best over the years. If you've picked up this book, chances are that you're a person who is interested in taking charge of your health, and this book is meant for you.

While we hope that you will benefit from our advice in this guide, this book isn't meant to substitute for seeing an eye doctor. A single book can never cover all that medical science knows today about eye health, and your eyes won't always behave according to the guidelines printed in a book. Because everyone's eyes are unique, seeing an eye doctor who can examine you and tell you what's important in your situation is extremely valuable when it comes to your eye care. We hope that our book will be a user-friendly reference guide to aid you as you navigate your way around this all-important medical territory.

Jennifer S. Weizer, M.D.
Joshua Stein, M.D., M.S.

1

How the Eye Works

The eye is an amazing sensory organ. The human eye is capable of seeing a candle flame from more than 30 miles away, and identifying objects as small as a piece of hair on a tabletop. Not only do we use our eyes to see objects near and far, our eyes enable us to see thousands of different colors, visualize objects in three dimensions, and detect even the slightest movements.

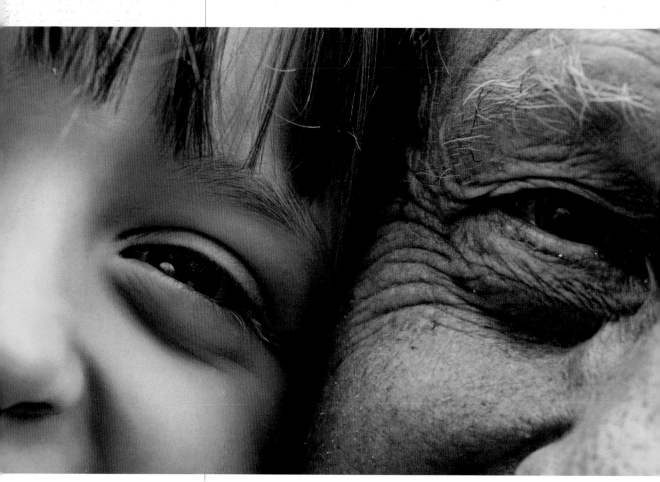

Overview of the eye

At birth, the human eye is approximately 1.6 to 1.7 cm in size. The eye grows rapidly over the first three years of life and reaches its full size, roughly 1 in. (2.5 cm) in diameter, by age 13. The eye is nearly spherical in shape. Despite its small size, the eye is a complex organ. To achieve clear vision, all the structures of the eye must be functioning properly, enabling the eye to capture light, bring it into focus, and relay messages back to the brain to make sense of visual stimuli.

Cornea

The cornea is located in the front of the eye and is a transparent structure whose main function is to focus light on the retina. When light goes through the cornea, it gets refracted or bent in a way so that it can be sharply focused on the retina.

Sclera

The sclera is the white part of the eye that makes up the eye wall. It provides structural support for all of the contents within the eye.

Conjunctiva

The conjunctiva is a thin layer of tissue on the inner surfaces of the eyelids and overlies the sclera in the front of the eye. It contains mucous-secreting cells. Its main function is to help keep the eye well lubricated.

Iris

The iris is the colored part of the eye situated between the cornea and the lens. The color of the iris is determined by its level of pigmentation. People with blue eyes have less pigment in their iris than those with

THE FRONT OF THE EYE

Incoming light enters the eye through the cornea. The cornea helps bend the rays of light so they can come to a sharp focus on the retina. Next the light goes through the pupil on its way back to the retina. The iris (the colored part of the eye) is responsible for blocking extraneous light from entering the pupil. The sclera is the white matter that keeps the other components in place. The conjunctiva contains cells that secrete moisture.

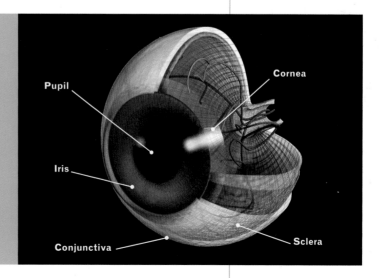

Pupil

Cornea

Iris

Conjunctiva

Sclera

brown eyes. The main purpose of the iris is to control the amount of light that enters the eye by blocking extraneous light from entering through the pupil.

Pupil

The pupil is the black spot in the center of the iris. Light goes through the pupil on its way to the retina. In dark settings, the pupil expands so that more light can enter the eye. In the presence of bright light, the size of the pupil gets smaller to prevent too much light from entering through the eye to the retina.

The size of the pupil can be affected by the use of various legal and illegal drugs. For example, persons who are ingesting cocaine often have dilated pupils, and individuals taking heroin usually have smaller than normal pupils.

Aqueous humor

The aqueous humor is the fluid in the front of the eye. Its function is to carry nutrients to the cornea and the lens and to remove waste products from the inside of the front of the eye.

Lens

The lens is located in the middle of the eye. Along with the cornea, it is responsible for focusing light on the retina. The lens comprises hundreds of thousands of tiny lens fibrils arranged in an orderly fashion so that light can penetrate through the lens undisturbed on its way to the retina. As a person gets older, the lens can become cloudy and develop into a cataract.

Vitreous humor

The large compartment of the eye between the lens and the retina is called the vitreous cavity. It is filled with a clear material called vitreous humor that has the consistency of jelly. The main purpose of the vitreous cavity is to help the eye maintain its normal shape and to provide a clear pathway so that light going through the eye can be focused on the retina.

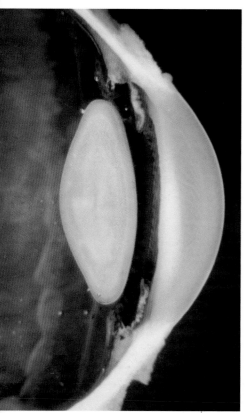

Cross-sectional view of the eye showing the cornea on the right (pale blue) and the lens in the center (yellow).

The vitreous humor makes up approximately 80 percent of the volume of the eyeball.

Retina

The retina is an important structure that absorbs and processes the light that enters the eye. If the eye is thought of as operating like a camera, the retina would be the film that captures each image the eye views.

The retina contains millions of photoreceptors called rods and cones. Most photoreceptor cells are rods, which are predominantly located in the peripheral retina. Rods function mainly at night; they are important for night vision and the detection of motion. The majority of photoreceptor cells in the center of the retina (the macula) are cones. The cones function predominantly in bright light settings and are responsible for color vision and fine vision.

Optic nerve

The optic nerve, or second cranial nerve, is an important structure that carries signals from the retina to the brain so they can be interpreted. It is composed of over one million axons, which carry visual information to different parts of the brain.

Macula

The macula is the central portion of the retina. This structure is very important for clear, distinct central vision. Common eye conditions that can cause damage to the macula include age-related macular degeneration and swelling of the macula caused by diabetic retinopathy. Damage to the macula from any cause often leads to a considerable decline in one's central vision.

Fovea

The fovea is a small depressed pit located in the center of the macula. This structure contains only cones. The fovea is where the sharpest vision takes place.

Even if all the structures in the eyeball are working properly, if the optic nerve is impaired, visual information entering the eye won't be transmitted to the brain, and the effect will be blindness.

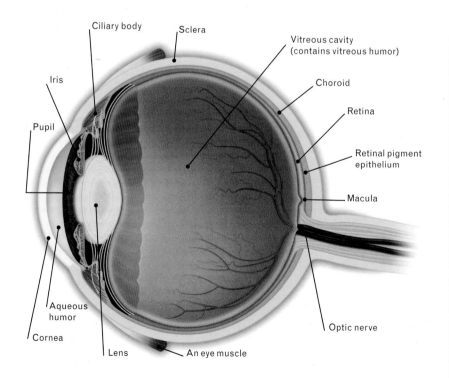

The lens helps bring light to focus on the retina. The light then travels through the vitreous cavity to the retina, and then the optic nerve transmits the signal to the brain.

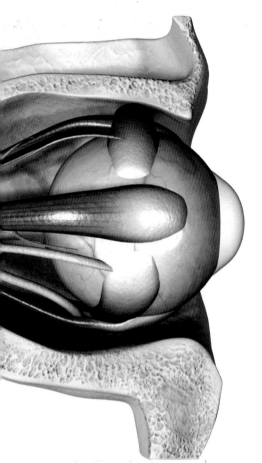

Choroid

The choroid is a vascular tissue located between the retinal pigment epithelium (see below) and the back wall of the eye. Its main function is to carry nutrients to the retina and the retinal pigment epithelium. The choroid also contains a pigment called melanin, which absorbs any extraneous light that would interfere with the image the eye is transmitting to the brain.

Retinal pigment epithelium

The retinal pigment epithelium is located directly behind the retina and in front of the choroid. This structure has several important functions, which include providing support to the photoreceptors and cleaning up any degenerated photoreceptors.

Eye muscles

There are six muscles that are attached to the outer surface of the eye wall of each eye. The muscles from both eyes work together so that both eyes are simultaneously viewing the same object. The eye muscles can move the eyes precisely enough to enable a person to quickly focus from one object to another during tasks such as reading and driving.

The eyeball is located in the center of the bony orbit. Eye muscles attach to the eyeball and help the eye move in different directions.

Eyelids

The upper and lower eyelids are composed of a thin layer of skin on the outer surface and moist conjunctiva on the inner surface. They function to protect the eyes by blinking to prevent debris from getting in the way of light entering into the eye.

Orbit

The orbit is the pocket of tissue that each eyeball sits in. Its walls are formed by seven different facial bones. In the center of the orbit sits each eyeball. Surrounding the eyeball within the orbit are muscles, nerves, blood vessels, fat, and lacrimal drainage system structures. The optic nerve exits the back of the orbit and carries visual information back to the brain.

The human eye spontaneously blinks, on average, 15 to 20 times per minute, which translates into nearly 30,000 blinks daily.

Lacrimal drainage system

The lacrimal drainage system is responsible for the production of tears, the distribution of tears over the surface of the eye, and the removal of any excess tears.

Lacrimal gland is a structure located in the upper outer portion of the orbit (eye socket). The lacrimal gland is important for producing the tears that bathe the surface of the eye.

Puncta are small holes that allow tears to drain from the eyes into the nose. The inner third of the upper and lower eyelid of each eye contains a punctum.

Nasolacrimal sac is a pouch situated under the skin between the eye and the nose that collects the tears from the eye and makes sure they continue to flow down into the nose.

Nasolacrimal duct is a tube situated under the skin that carries the tears from the nasolacrimal sac down to the nose.

Tear film bathes the front surface of the eye, providing nourishment to the cornea, preventing dryness, and removing surface debris. Tears have three components: water, lipid, and mucus. The tears are produced by the lacrimal gland. After bathing the front surface of the eye, the tears enter the puncta and travel through the nasolacrimal sac and duct to eventually drain into the nose and down the throat. The tears coat the front surface of the eye, but there is no direct connection to the inside of the eye, which is filled with aqueous humor and vitreous humor.

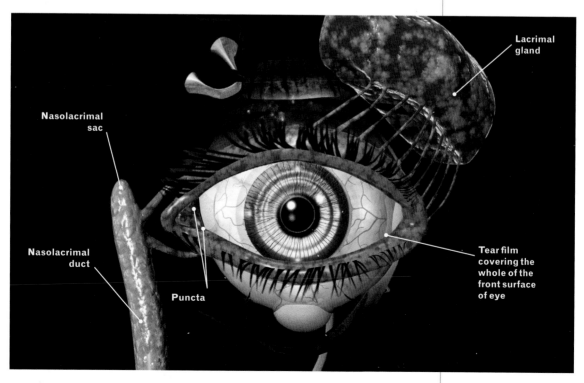

Lacrimal gland

Nasolacrimal sac

Nasolacrimal duct

Puncta

Tear film covering the whole of the front surface of eye

How we see

When you look at an object, some of the rays of light that illuminate it are reflected off the object and into your eye. The first structure of the eye the light rays reach is the cornea. When the rays go through the cornea, they are refracted, or bent slightly, and are brought into focus. After exiting through the cornea, the rays continue traveling deeper into the eye. The next structures that the rays of light encounter are the iris and the pupil. The iris blocks light rays from penetrating deeper into the eye, and only the rays of light that enter through the pupil are processed. The size of the pupil varies depending on the brightness of the environment. On a bright, sunny day, the pupil contracts, restricting excess light from entering the eye. But when it is dark, the pupil expands to maximize the amount of light entering the back of the eye.

The next structure that the rays of light reach is the lens. The lens refracts or bends the rays of light some more to bring them into focus. The rays then travel through the vitreous cavity and are brought further into focus on the retina. Different photoreceptors in the retina are stimulated by different wavelengths of light. The activated cells in the retina send their signals to the optic nerve, which in turn transmits the signal to the brain. The brain processes and makes sense of the signals.

Visual acuity

Visual acuity is a measurement of how well the eye is able to see fine detail. For infants, who cannot yet speak, visual acuity is determined by the child's ability to fixate on an object and follow it with her eyes. Visual acuity in young children can be measured by showing them pictures at varying distances. For older children and adults, visual acuity is routinely tested by using a Snellen chart, which contains letters of the alphabet of different sizes. One stands at a fixed distance from the vision chart, and the smaller the letters one can read, the better the visual acuity is. In tests of visual acuity, one eye is usually covered so that each eye is tested individually. Visual acuity can be tested with optical correction (eyeglasses or contact lenses) to help determine whether corrective devices can improve how well the eye can see.

20/20 vision

The results of the visual acuity test are presented as a fraction. The numerator of the fraction is the distance measured in feet that you are from the vision chart when reading the finest print you

Objects are illuminated by the sun and other light sources. Some of the light rays bounce off the object and enter into the eye.

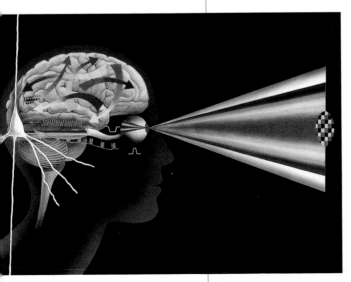

are capable of seeing on the chart. The denominator of the fraction is the distance in feet that a person with normal vision can stand away from the chart and read the same letters. For example, if your vision is 20/200, the smallest letters of the chart that you are capable of reading when you stand 20 feet away from it can be read by a person with normal vision who stands 200 feet away from it. In this system, perfect vision is 20/20.

Color vision

The retina contains several specialized cells called photoreceptors that absorb different wavelengths of light. There are two types of photoreceptor cells: rods and cones. Rods detect objects in dimly lit environments, but do not detect color. This is why when it is dark, it is difficult to see the color of objects. Alternatively, cone cells respond best in bright settings. There are three types of cone cells: S cones, M cones, and L cones. Each of these types responds best to different wavelengths of light. The S cones respond best to short wavelengths of light, the M cones to medium wavelengths of light, and the L cones to long wavelengths of light. The human retina can perceive wavelengths of light in the range of 350 to 750 nanometers. Objects that are blue or violet absorb all the wavelengths of light except short wavelengths of light in the 400 to 500 nanometer range. These short wavelengths are reflected off objects and stimulate the S cones in the retina.

Ultraviolet wavelengths are invisible to the human eye without the aid of special detection devices, but some birds and fish can detect wavelengths in the ultraviolet range.

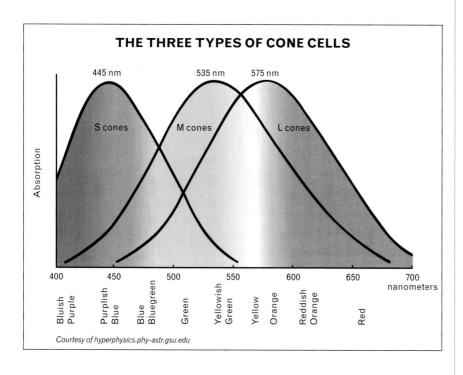

THE THREE TYPES OF CONE CELLS

Courtesy of hyperphysics.phy-astr.gsu.edu

An example of one of the Ishihara color test pictures. Individuals who are color blind have difficulty seeing the embedded number.

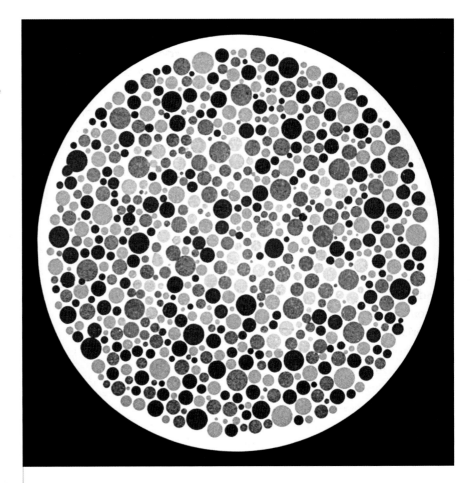

Similarly, objects that are orange or red absorb all the wavelengths of light besides long wavelengths of light in the 600 to 700 nanometer range, which are reflected off the object and detected by the L-cone cells. The brain combines the signals from the different photoreceptor cells in the retina that have been stimulated to perceive color. Wavelengths that are just below the spectrum of visible light that humans are capable of seeing are ultraviolet, and those that are just above the spectrum of visible light are infrared.

The vast majority of people with color blindness can see color, but they have difficulty discriminating between different hues or shades.

Approximately 5 to 8 percent of males and less than 1 percent of females are color blind. This condition is usually genetically inherited. The most common form of color blindness is red-green color blindness. In this condition, there is a defect in one of the types of cone receptors. For example, the M-cone cells, which normally respond to wavelengths of light in the green spectrum, may instead respond to wavelengths of light that are closer to the red spectrum.

There are different ways to test for color blindness. A commonly used test is the Ishihara color test. This test consists of a series of pictures composed of many dots. The background of the picture is made up of dots of one color shade, and embedded within the picture are dots of another color shade that form a number. Persons who have normal color vision have no difficulty in seeing the embedded number in the picture, but those with color blindness struggle to identify the number. In addition to genetically inherited color blindness, certain disorders of the optic nerve can also lead to a reduction in the ability to perceive colors.

Visual field

The field of vision is the amount of peripheral or side vision an eye is capable of when looking straight ahead. A healthy eye is capable of seeing 60 degrees inward (toward the nose), 100 degrees outward (away from the nose), 60 degrees above and 75 degrees below the midline. Certain eye diseases, such as glaucoma, droopy eyelids, and stroke can all reduce a person's peripheral vision.

Peripheral vision can be measured using various methods. The most common methods include confrontational visual field testing, Goldmann perimetry, and standard automated perimetry. In performing visual field testing, each eye is usually tested separately, with a cover placed over the eye that is not being tested.

Below is an example of a printout of a visual field test with a normal result. The center of the printout is where the clearest, sharpest vision is located. Note the black spot that is present just off the center of the printout.

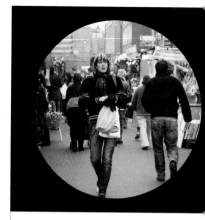

Normal field of vision.

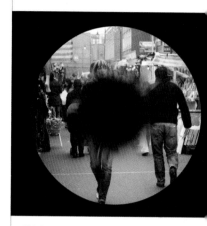

With macular degeneration, one can develop a loss of central vision.

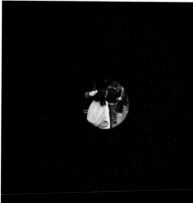

With advanced glaucoma much of the peripheral vision is lost.

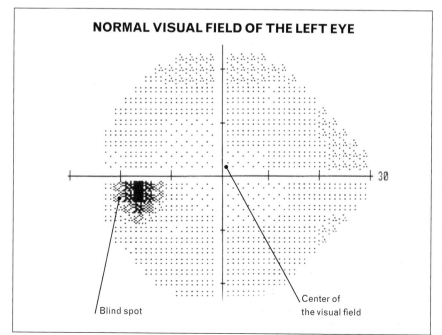

NORMAL VISUAL FIELD OF THE LEFT EYE

30

Blind spot

Center of
the visual field

This represents the blind spot. Every eye has a blind spot, which is the location where light entering the eye is focused on the optic nerve and not the retina. Since the optic nerve is incapable of absorbing the rays of light entering the eye (its function is to transmit the signals from the retina to the brain), a person cannot see an object situated in her blind spot.

We usually do not notice that we have a blind spot because we view objects using both of our eyes simultaneously. An object located in the blind spot of one eye would not be in the blind spot of the second eye, which is able to see the object.

Diseases can affect different structures in the eye or the brain. Depending on which structures are involved, the effect on the field of vision will vary. For example, a condition such as age-related macular degeneration usually damages the cells in the center of the retina, resulting in the loss of central vision. Since the cells located outside the center of the retina are not affected, patients with this condition usually have normal peripheral vision. Alternatively, most forms of glaucoma cause damage to the cells carrying information from the periphery, producing loss of peripheral vision. As the disease becomes advanced, patients with glaucoma tend to develop tunnel vision, in which they can see objects only in the center of their visual field.

OPTICAL ILLUSION

It is a myth that everyone who is legally blind knows Braille. It is estimated that only 10 percent of blind people know Braille. Fortunately, many people who are legally blind are able to use magnifying lenses or other optical devices to help them see well enough to care for themselves.

Legal blindness

In the United States, Canada, and many European countries, the definition of legal blindness is vision with best-correction (using eyeglasses or contact lenses, if necessary) of 20/200 or worse in the better-seeing eye or a visual field (peripheral vision) of 20 degrees or less remaining. What this means is that when wearing glasses or contact lenses, if the best you are able to see from either eye is the large E on the eye chart, you would meet the criteria for legal blindness. In Australia, a person who is legally blind may have a

TIPS ON SELECTING AN EYE CARE PROVIDER

- Review the diplomas and credentials of the provider to make sure he or she is properly trained.
- Ask the eye care professional whether he or she has received specific training to perform the types of services you require.
- If you require a surgical procedure, inquire about the number of times the provider has performed the specific procedure you are seeking.
- Get recommendations from family members or friends you know who have had the procedure you need or from your primary care provider.

visual acuity of 6/60 or less (in the better-seeing eye, wearing glasses or contact lenses), a visual field of less than 10 degrees, or both.

Finally, it is important to realize that the level of vision for legal blindness is different from the level of vision required to drive a car. In the United States, the level of vision necessary for driving varies from one state to another. The International Academy of Low Vision Specialists provides the criteria that each state requires.

In Canada, if your visual acuity is worse than 20/50, you are disqualified from obtaining a driver's license or are restricted to daytime driving only. Please refer to the Canadian National Institute for the Blind (CNIB) for further information. Australian readers should check with their state roads and traffic authority for the relevant regulations.

> Legal blindness is not the same as a complete inability to see any light. In fact, many individuals who are legally blind are able to see well enough to perform many activities.

Types of eye care providers

When you have a problem with your vision and are seeking assistance from an eye care professional, it is important that you go to someone who is qualified and trained to address your specific eye care needs.

Ophthalmologist

Ophthalmologists are physicians. They have college and medical school degrees, each typically requiring four years of full-time study and at least three additional years of training after medical school in the medical and surgical treatment of patients with eye conditions.

Optometrist

Optometrists are eye care professionals who have completed four years of college and four years of optometry school. They receive formal training in prescribing eyeglasses and contact lenses and in diagnosing eye problems. In some U.S. states they can prescribe medications to treat minor ocular conditions; however, they are not allowed to perform eye surgery.

Optician

Opticians are eye care professionals who are trained to fit patients with eyeglasses.

Optometrist using equipment to check a patient's eyeglasses prescription.

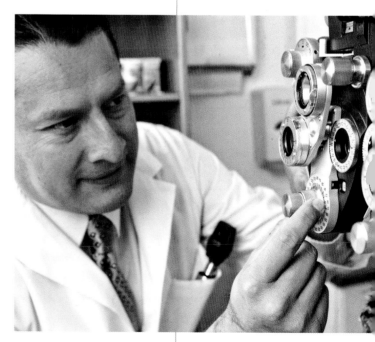

They check the frames of glasses to make sure they fit properly. They are not allowed to prescribe medications or to perform surgical procedures.

Orthoptist

Orthoptists are eye care providers who specialize in caring for patients with problems with eye movement or eye alignment. They frequently assist ophthalmologists in caring for patients with crossed eyes (strabismus) or double vision (diplopia). They use prisms and other optical aids to help align the eyes. They do not prescribe medications or perform surgical procedures.

The qualifications and training of these types of eye care professionals in Australia and New Zealand are slightly different but comparable to those in the United States.

TYPES OF EYE CARE PROVIDERS	
OPHTHALMOLOGIST (PHYSICIAN)	• Performs routine eye examinations • Diagnoses and treats ocular diseases, such as cataracts and glaucoma • Diagnoses systemic conditions that affect the eyes, such as diabetic retinopathy • Prescribes eyeglasses, contact lenses, low-vision aids and medications • Performs surgical procedures, such as cataract surgery or refractive surgery
OPTOMETRIST	• Performs routine eye examinations • Diagnoses ocular diseases, such as cataracts and glaucoma • Diagnoses systemic conditions that affect the eyes, such as diabetic retinopathy • Prescribes eyeglasses, contact lenses, and low-vision aids • Does not perform eye surgery
OPTICIAN	• Adjusts and fits eyeglasses • Takes facial measurements to determine appropriately sized frames • Dispenses eyewear • Makes sure clients know how to care for their eyewear • Does not write prescriptions for glasses or contact lenses • Does not examine the eyes or diagnose or treat eye diseases

Routine eye examination

A routine eye examination usually begins with your eye care professional obtaining a thorough history, enabling her to learn all about your eyes. Some of the types of questions you will be asked include whether or not your eyes are bothering you; whether you have any known eye diseases, such as cataracts or glaucoma; or if any members of your family have any eye conditions. If you are known to have a particular ocular condition, it can be very useful to bring to your appointment copies of records revealing the results of ocular diagnostic tests and treatments you have previously undergone from other eye care providers who have cared for you.

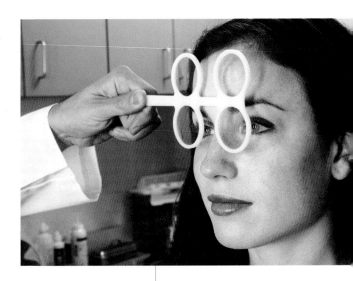

Before being examined by your eye doctor, you'll be asked about your eye history as well as your medical history.

Other questions you may be asked by your eye doctor include whether your eyes have ever been injured or if you have ever undergone a surgical procedure. The eye care provider will want to know if you wear eyeglasses or contact lenses. If you have a copy of your most recent eyeglass or contact lens prescription, that would be useful to bring to your appointment. You may also be asked about your nonocular medical history, because several common medical conditions, such as diabetes mellitus, hypertension (high blood pressure), and thyroid disease, can damage eyes over time. The eye care provider will want to know about all of the prescription and over-the-counter medications, vitamins, and herbal supplements you take, since some products can be beneficial or detrimental to the health of your eye. Other questions you will probably be asked include whether or not you smoke cigarettes or use illicit drugs. It is important to answer these questions truthfully to provide your eye doctor with a complete medical history.

Schedule for eye examinations

The frequency with which you should have your eyes examined depends on a variety of factors, including your age, your medical history, whether you have any known ocular conditions, and your family history of ocular conditions.

A recommended examination schedule, from the Kellogg Eye Center at the University of Michigan School of Medicine, is shown on page 25. It outlines how frequently individuals of different ages should have an eye examination, and the table on page 24 provides a list of individuals with specific medical or ocular conditions who are at increased risk of experiencing

---

QUESTIONS TO ASK YOUR EYE DOCTOR

- **What tests will be performed on my eyes at today's visit?**

- **Are there any new problems you are noticing with my eyes since my last visit to see you?**

- **Has my vision changed in either eye from the last time I came to see you?**

- **Do I have any eye conditions that can run in the family, and if so, should I tell my parents, siblings, or children to have their eyes examined?**

- **If there are any problems with my eyes, what are the best ways to manage them?**

HIGH-RISK GROUPS THAT MAY REQUIRE MORE FREQUENT EYE EXAMINATIONS

CHILDREN	
	Premature newborns Especially those with a low birth weight and those requiring supplemental oxygen
	History of maternal infection or substance abuse at time of childbirth
	Fetal distress during labor
	Family history of congenital eye conditions Examples include: strabismus (crossed eyes), amblyopia (lazy eye), cataracts, retinoblastoma
	Medical condition that can affect eyesight Examples include: sickle cell disease, diabetes mellitus, diseases of the central nervous system, certain genetic or metabolic conditions
	Strong eyeglass prescriptions for myopia (nearsightedness), hyperopia (farsightedness), or astigmatism
	Anisometropia (large difference in eyeglass prescription between the two eyes)
	Ocular conditions such as congenital cataracts, glaucoma, strabismus, amblyopia
	Any previous eye surgery
ADULTS	**Diabetes mellitus**
	Hypertension (high blood pressure)
	HIV/AIDS
	Family or personal history of glaucoma or age-related macular degeneration
	Contact lens wearers
	Previous eye surgery
	Previous eye injury
	Medical condition that can affect the eye (see chapter 4)
	Use of a medication known to affect eyes (see chapter 5)

Courtesy of Kellogg Eye Center at the University of Michigan School of Medicine

damage to their eyes and thus should be followed closely by an eye care professional.

Vision check

A standard eye examination in adults usually begins with a check of the vision in each eye. To check distance vision, one eye is covered while the other reads the letters on a chart. This test will determine how well you can see without corrective lenses or with your current prescription lenses. If you cannot see clearly, the eye care provider may perform a refraction: he or she tries out different combinations of lenses to determine whether a new prescription can help you to see more clearly. After your distance vision is checked, your near or reading vision will be assessed. Often, you will be given a card that has small print and be asked to hold it at the distance you would normally hold a newspaper or magazine and read the smallest print you can make out. If you are unable to see the small print clearly, you may require corrective lenses for reading. Measurements will be taken to determine the appropriate strength of the reading prescription that will optimize your near vision.

Encourage a friend or loved one to go with you to your appointment. Having another set of ears around is useful to help you remember some of the information that your eye doctor is explaining to you about your eye condition.

Alignment and peripheral vision

Next tests will be conducted to observe whether your eyes are correctly aligned with one another and whether they can move in different directions of gaze (up, down, right, left, and toward your nose). A check of your pupils will be performed by asking you to gaze across the room while the provider shines a bright light into one eye. When your eyes are functioning properly, the bright light will stimulate both of your pupils to contract.

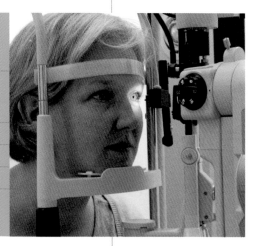

An eye care provider examining the eye using a slit lamp.

HOW OFTEN TO HAVE YOUR EYES EXAMINED

AGE	FREQUENCY
0 to 6 months	At least once by an ophthalmologist or a pediatrician
6 months to 18 years	Every 2–4 years
19 to 39 years	Every 3–5 years
40 to 64 years	Every 2–4 years
65 or older	Every 1–2 years

Courtesy of the Kellogg Eye Center at the University of Michigan School of Medicine

QUESTIONS TO ASK YOUR EYE DOCTOR

- **Does your office have any brochures that describe the conditions affecting my eyes?**

- **If I have any questions after my visit, when is a good time to contact you?**

- **When should I return to see you again for another examination?**

Another commonly performed test checks your peripheral vision. As outlined earlier in the chapter, there are different ways to perform visual field testing. A simple way to check the peripheral vision is to cover one eye and stare straight ahead. The examiner will hold up fingers in your peripheral field of vision and ask you to state the number of fingers you see. The same test is then performed on the other eye.

Slit-lamp

An effective way for an eye care provider to examine your eyes is to use a slit-lamp. This machine lets the examiner focus on different structures in the front and back of the eye to check whether or not the eye is functioning properly. The examiner can adjust the intensity of the light and the level of magnification. You will be asked to keep your chin on the chin rest and to lean forward. If you feel uncomfortable with how your head is positioned during the examination, tell the examiner and she can adjust the equipment for better comfort. The examiner will check all of the structures in the front of the eye. Next you will be given an anesthetic eyedrop that temporarily numbs the front surface of the eye and also a substance called fluorescein that coats the front surface of the eye and lights up when exposed to a light with a blue filter. The anesthetic eyedrop and the fluorescein allow the provider to check the intraocular pressure in each eye. For the check of the eye pressure, you will need to keep your eyes wide open and breathe normally. A device attached to the slit-lamp called a tonometer will be brought up to the front surface of your eye and will measure the level of pressure in each eye. Some providers check eye pressure using a puff of air on the surface of the eye.

Slit-lamp examination of a patient's right eye.

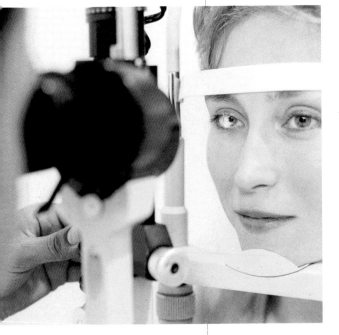

Dilating the pupil

A full eye examination involves dilating the eyes so the eye care provider can obtain a detailed look at the structures in the back of the eye. Often medications such as phenylephrine and tropicamide eyedrops are used to dilate the pupil. It can take up to 30 minutes for the dilating drops to act. Your vision will be blurry temporarily as a result. The time your eyes remain dilated depends on factors including the type and strength of the dilating drops and the color of your iris. For most patients, the eyes stay dilated for 4 to 8 hours. If they remain dilated for more than 24 hours, tell your eye care provider. During a dilated eye examination, the eye care professional will examine the lens, the vitreous humor, the retina, the blood vessels, and the optic nerve.

A routine complete eye examination is different for infants and children. It is advisable to have your child's eyes examined regularly if eye problems are prevalent in your family. As a final note to add, patients with specific ocular conditions such as glaucoma, diabetic retinopathy, or age-related macular degeneration may need to undergo further diagnostic procedures not covered in this section. Please consult your eye doctor for further advice if you are worried about any of these conditions.

ROUTINE EYE EXAMINATION	
TEST	FUNCTION
VISION CHECK	Determines whether you are able to see clearly to perform activities such as driving and reading.
REFRACTION	Determines whether you require corrective lenses to improve your distance or near vision.
OCULAR MOTILITY	Determines whether the eyes are able to move properly in all directions of gaze.
PUPIL EXAMINATION	Determines the responses of the pupils to bright light to see whether the optic nerves are functioning properly.
VISUAL FIELD	Checks your peripheral vision.
SLIT-LAMP EXAMINATION	Allows the eye care professional to obtain a detailed view of all of the structures in the front and back of the eye.
TONOMETRY	Checks the intraocular pressure in each of the eyes; elevated intraocular pressure is a risk factor for glaucoma.
DILATED FUNDOSCOPY	Dilating eyedrops cause the pupils to enlarge, which allows the eye care professional to obtain a better view of the retina, blood vessels, and optic nerves.

2

Perfectly Clear

While a lucky minority of people will never need to wear glasses or contact lenses, many of us must rely on some type of vision correction to optimize our vision. Advances in today's technology are making glasses and contact lenses easier and more comfortable to wear, while refractive surgery is becoming an increasingly popular option for many people.

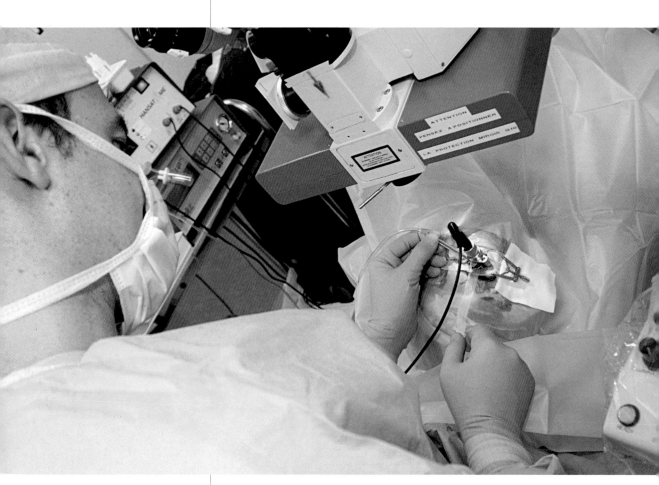

Optimizing your vision

Imagine that a perfectly shaped eyeball is exactly round, like a Ping-Pong ball, allowing you to see objects clearly, both far away and up close, without the help of glasses. For many of us, however, our eyeballs develop just slightly imperfectly, so that they are not exactly round. Even if our eyeballs vary just a fraction of a millimeter from perfect spheres, the result is that we may be nearsighted, farsighted, or have astigmatism. For these reasons, you may need glasses or contact lenses to see your very best.

Nearsightedness

Do you work at your computer with ease but have trouble making out the details of objects far away? If you need glasses to see things at a distance, there is a good chance that you are nearsighted. Nearsightedness, or myopia, affects about 25 percent of the population. Distant objects seem blurry if you aren't wearing glasses or contact lenses, while objects up close, at reading distance, are clearer. There are several causes for nearsightedness, including the shape of your cornea, the placement and shape of your eye's natural lens, and having a longer eyeball than normal. Because of one or more of these factors, the image a distant object forms in the eye is located in front of, rather than exactly on, the retina, so a blurry image is sent to the brain.

Farsightedness

Do you find yourself squinting at books, even though you can read signs from a distance? Farsightedness, or hyperopia, affects about 10 percent of the adult population. Though many children are farsighted, they often grow out of this naturally as they reach adulthood. As we age, however, farsightedness makes it harder to see distant objects as well as near ones.

The factors that contribute to farsightedness are parallel to those in nearsightedness, namely the shape of the cornea, the placement and shape

TEST YOUR
Eye Q:

True or False?
Each of us has a dominant eye and a non-dominant eye, similar in concept to being right- or left-handed?

True

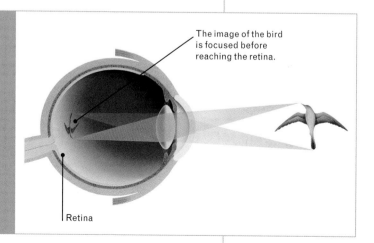

MYOPIA

Nearsightedness: in this diagram we can see what happens to the vision in a nearsighted eye. The image of a distant object is focused too far in front of the retina, rather than precisely on the retina itself. This means that a blurry image is sent to the brain and the person will experience difficulty in focusing on the faraway object.

In a farsighted eye the image is focused too far behind the retina.

The image of the bird is focused before reaching the retina.

Retina

of the eye's lens, and a shorter eyeball than usual. In cases of farsightedness, however, the image a distant object forms in your eye is located behind, rather than exactly on, your retina, which again results in a blurry image being sent to the visual part of your brain.

The eye's natural lens accommodates, or changes, its shape, so that we can see things up close. This accommodative ability is lost as we get older.

Presbyopia

Have you ever wondered why some older people need to hold books and newspapers farther away from their eyes to be able to read the small print? Presbyopia, or loss of ability to accommodate due to age, is the reason. While we are young, the eye's lens is able to change its shape, or accommodate, to focus on objects that are close to the eye. As we reach middle age, the ciliary body inside our eyes begins to lose its ability to contract, and the lens becomes thicker and stiffer. Our eyes are less able to accommodate, and it becomes harder to see objects without using a corrective device.

Astigmatism

A normal cornea is shaped like a partial sphere in which every axis, or direction, is equally curved. The eye's natural lens also has a curvature that is usually equal in all directions. For people with astigmatism, some axes of the cornea or the lens may be steeper than others. The image does not fall exactly on the retina and, as with nearsightedness and farsightedness, that image is seen by the brain as blurry. It is common to experience astigmatism along with nearsightedness or farsightedness.

OPTICAL ILLUSION

Many people wonder if eye exercises can reduce their need for glasses or contact lenses. In the vast majority of cases, eye exercises do not help. It's better to wear glasses or contact lenses if they help you to achieve your optimum vision.

Glasses

Glasses correct most vision problems and are the safest of the available options. Glasses change the way your eye focuses so that, for nearsighted people, an image that would have been located in front of your retina is now located directly on the retina, sending a clear picture to your brain. Likewise, in farsightedness, glasses focus the image on your retina rather than behind it, giving you a clearer image. Glasses correct most cases of astigmatism, too. If you experience presbyopia, reading or bifocal glasses give you focusing power that makes up for accommodation lost naturally with age, which will improve your near vision.

What to expect when you get glasses

With all the different types of glasses on the market, how do you know which will suit your eyes best? The answer depends on the particular vision problems you have, since each particular style is suited to a different combination of issues.

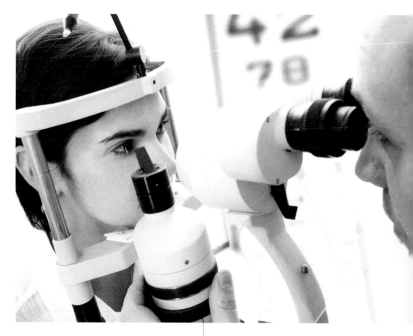

The process of being fit for glasses has several steps. First your eye doctor will perform an examination to determine the prescription that will give you optimum vision. The doctor may measure your current glasses, if you normally wear glasses, as a starting point to see if that prescription needs to be adjusted. After you receive the prescription, you can take it to an optician to choose a new frame. After you decide on the frames, your optician will use your glasses prescription to order and fit your frame and lenses.

The slit lamp examination allows your optometrist or ophthalmologist to get a close look at the internal structures of the eye.

Finding a qualified optician is a very important step in a successful fitting. Sometimes adjustments to how the lenses are made will correct or alleviate particular problems. Also, certain frames may suit certain prescriptions best, and not all glasses prescriptions are appropriate for all frames. A good optician can give you advice on which frames or lens types will work best for your own refractive needs.

Glasses remain the healthiest and safest way to correct refractive error, since there is no risk of infection or allergy from wearing them. Glasses are

CARE INSTRUCTIONS FOR EYEWEAR

- Wash your lenses daily with mild soap and water or commercially available lens cleaner to remove oil and dirt.
- Dry your lenses with a soft, clean cloth.
- Do not clean your lenses with tissues or other paper products.
- Do not expose your eyewear to extreme temperature conditions (for example, do not leave your glasses on the dashboard of a car).
- Avoid laying your lenses face down.
- Never use household cleaners that contain ammonia or bleach to clean your lenses, as these can cause damage to the material.
- Store your eyewear in a case when not in use.

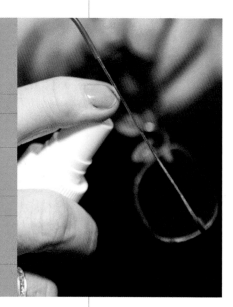

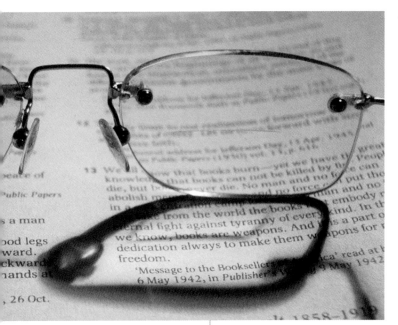

easy to replace if your prescription changes over time, and they can also make a fashion statement. With the wide variety of frames and lens materials on the market, it is possible for almost everyone who needs their vision corrected to find the right pair of glasses.

Single vision

Single vision glasses have one strength in each lens, so each of your eyes will be corrected for either nearsightedness or farsightedness, as well as any possible astigmatism.

In this pair of bifocal glasses, we can see the dividing line between the two segments of the lens.

Bifocal

Bifocal glasses correct distance vision in the top part of each lens and near correction in the bottom part of each lens, and the two segments are divided by a line. Bifocal glasses are typically worn by presbyopic adults or, more rarely, by children who have trouble with accommodation.

Trifocal

Trifocal glasses have three segments: distance correction in the top part of each lens, intermediate distance correction in the middle part of each lens, and near correction in the bottom part of each lens. Each of the three segments is divided by a line. The intermediate distance segment of the lens is often useful for computer work, for reading instruments on a car dashboard, or for reading music on a music stand, for example.

OPTICAL ILLUSION

Many people think that prescription reading glasses are better for their eyes. In fact, over-the-counter reading glasses work just as well.

Progressive

Progressive lenses, on the other hand, have distance correction in the top part of each lens and near correction in the bottom, but instead of having a line between those two segments, the strength gradually changes between the top and bottom, without a visible line.

That middle area of gradual change in lens strength can be used for intermediate distance vision. It may be cosmetically appealing not to have a visible line in your lenses, but the area of intermediate distance correction and near vision correction is smaller in a progressive lens than in a bifocal or trifocal lens, so it may be slightly more difficult to find the "sweet spot" for clearest vision at intermediate and close-up distances. Also, there is more distortion when looking to the right and left through the side areas than with bifocal and trifocal lenses.

Over-the-counter reading glasses

If you are lucky enough not to need glasses to see things at a distance but do need help to read, over-the-counter reading glasses are widely available without a prescription. The strength that works best for you will depend both on your age and on how well your eyes accommodate (how the natural lenses inside your eyes change their shape so that you can see up close), as well as whether or not you have had cataract surgery. Younger people tend to need weaker reading glasses, while older people or those who have had cataract surgery need stronger ones. When deciding which over-the-counter reading glasses to buy, start by picking a pair from the rack in the store and then try to read a magazine or book to decide which strength will work best for you.

Eyeglass materials

Many years ago, lenses were made of glass, but today's plastic lenses are a much safer, lighter material. Lenses can be made out of regular plastic, high-index plastic, or polycarbonate.

High-index lenses are thinner and lighter than regular plastic lenses, so they may be especially helpful if you have a strong prescription that would require thick lenses if they were made of regular plastic. High-index lenses are slightly more shatter resistant than regular plastic lenses and have ultraviolet protection built in.

Polycarbonate lenses are lightweight and shatter resistant, and often used as sports eyewear and for children's glasses. Polycarbonate lenses are especially important for people with good vision in only one eye in order to protect that good eye from injury. They also have ultraviolet protection built into the lens.

Lens coatings

Various coatings are available for your lenses. Though some coatings may be expensive, sometimes they can be well worth the cost.

Ultraviolet coatings can be added to plastic lenses that are neither high index nor polycarbonate and so do not have ultraviolet protection already built into the lens.

Anti-glare coating is also often recommended, since it can actually improve vision in addition to preventing glare.

Scratch resistant coating is available for regular plastic lenses and is a practical addition.

Frames
The variety of available frames continues to grow, and plastic and metal frames are probably the most popular. Newer titanium frames are quite resistant to damage, and polycarbonate frames are a safe choice to use with polycarbonate lenses, especially if you play sports or have good vision in only one eye.

Safety first
Your eyes can be easily damaged in certain situations—during sports and around hazardous materials in particular. As most of this damage is difficult or impossible to reverse, taking care to prevent it from happening in the first place is the most sensible way to keep your eyes in top condition.

Glasses and sun protection
Wearing glasses that protect against ultraviolet rays is a good habit, whatever your age. Too much ultraviolet light exposure may increase the risk of developing cataract and macular degeneration later in life. For protection, look for ultraviolet protective coatings on prescription glasses or for sunglasses with ultraviolet protection. Ultraviolet protective coatings can be applied to regular plastic lenses, but high-index and polycarbonate lenses already have this protection built in. For sunglasses, look for a brand that states its lenses have ultraviolet protection, since this is more important for the health of your eyes than the actual tint of the sunglass lenses. If you want the tint of sunglasses with the convenience of not needing a separate pair of frames, you may want to consider photochromic or "transition" lenses. These lenses are clear in dim light conditions but darken in brighter lighting, such as when you go outside into bright sunlight. They can be made of regular plastic, high-index plastic, or polycarbonate and come in several different tints. Whether or not you would benefit from photochromic lenses as opposed to sunglasses is largely a matter of personal preference. Also note that hats with broad brims can protect your face and head from too much sun exposure and can also help protect your eyes from ultraviolet light.

---

5 THINGS TO LOOK FOR IN SUNGLASSES

1. When selecting a pair of sunglasses, it is important to make sure that they have ultraviolet protection to ensure the health and safety of your eyes.

2. Different color tints filter light in different ways. Gray tints are a good choice because they reduce glare without distorting color.

3. Choose a pair of sunglasses with large lenses to adequately cover your eyes, protecting them from ultraviolet light.

4. Make sure that the frame and lenses fit comfortably, particularly over the bridge of the nose.

5. Make sure that the hinges and nose piece feel sturdy and that the lenses are secure.

Safety glasses and eye protection

Safety glasses are strongly recommended whenever you perform a task in which there's even a small chance of an object hitting your eye, such as mowing the lawn, using a line lawn trimmer, using power tools, or hammering on metal. Eye injuries, particularly severe ones in which the eyeball is penetrated by a foreign object, can be very damaging and have long-term consequences for a person's vision.

Safety glasses are widely available at hardware stores. The most effective ones are shaped like goggles for more complete eye protection. People with good vision in only one eye should take special care not only to use safety glasses for dangerous tasks but also to wear glasses with polycarbonate lenses at all times.

Children and eye safety

Set a good example for your children by using safety glasses whenever appropriate and take special care to make sure that all the toys they play with are age-appropriate.

Encourage children to get into good eye care habits early to keep their eyes safe for life.

- Never let a child light fireworks or stand near someone who is lighting fireworks.
- Do not let a child near a lawnmower that is being operated, since flying rocks and debris can cause serious eye injuries.
- Keep household chemicals and sprays out of the children's reach.
- Be aware that many household objects, such as paper clips, fishing hooks, rubber bands, wire coat hangers, and elastic cords can cause serious eye injuries.
- Always provide schoolchildren, in particular, with protective goggles in shop classes or science labs.

The majority of serious eye injuries occur in people younger than 25 years old.

Sports safety

Both adults and children who wear glasses or contact lenses should use proper protective eyewear while playing sports. This can include shatter-resistant frames and polycarbonate lenses.

- Baseball players should wear a protective helmet with a polycarbonate face shield while batting.
- Hockey players should wear a protective helmet with a polycarbonate or wire face shield certified by the Hockey Equipment Certification

Council (HECC) in the United States or, in Canada, by the Canadian Standards Association (CSA).

- Sports goggles with polycarbonate lenses, which can be made with lens prescriptions, should be worn for basketball, soccer, tennis, and racketball.
- Boxing poses a serious threat for severe eye injury, and no adequate protection exists for this sport. If you have good vision in one eye only, carefully consider the risks of injury to your good eye before deciding whether or not to participate.

Contact lenses

If you prefer not to wear glasses, contact lenses are an alternative to consider. Contact lenses are thin disks made of plastic that are designed to cover the cornea, or the clear front part of your eyeball. They stay in position on the cornea because of surface tension, a force that causes the contact lens to adhere to the natural tear film on the surface of your eye. Like eyeglasses, contact lenses can correct nearsightedness, farsightedness, astigmatism, and presbyopia.

It is always best to get a proper contact lens fitting by a qualified eye doctor to make sure you can wear your contact lenses safely and comfortably. A contact lens prescription is not the same as a glasses prescription because, beyond specifying the vision correction needed, a contact lens prescription also specifies the curvature and diameter of the contact lens. Often, several fittings with various lenses are needed before a good fit is found, but having patience during this process can pay off since using your optimal contact lenses will maximize the safety and comfort of your eyes. Most people can wear contact lenses for vision correction, but you might not be a good candidate if:

Most people find it easy to wear contact lenses after some practice in handling and inserting them.

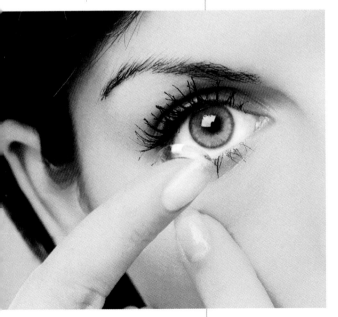

- you are prone to frequent eye infections or severe allergies, since you may notice that these symptoms worsen with lens wear.
- you have difficulty handling and cleaning contact lenses.

Soft contact lenses

Lenses come in a variety of materials. Soft disposable contact lenses are made to be worn for a certain length of time. Daily disposable soft contact lenses tend to be the most expensive, but because they are discarded each day, there is no need to buy and deal with cleaning products. Soft disposable contact lenses that are designed to be worn for 2-4 weeks before being discarded should be cleaned on a daily basis.

Soft disposable lenses are the most commonly prescribed lenses and range in recommended length of wear from one day to several weeks. These lenses are made of different types of plastics. Most recently, silicone hydrogel (a mixture of silicone with other plastics) has risen to the forefront of contact lens materials. Compared to older materials, silicone hydrogel allows more oxygen to penetrate the cornea, which is good for the health of your eyeball. These lenses tend to stay moister and are generally more comfortable than other types. They are also more resistant to the deposits of protein and debris that can accumulate on the surface.

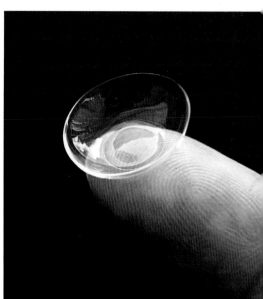

Soft disposable lenses can correct a small amount of astigmatism in addition to near or farsightedness. This is because the contact lens floats on the tear film and forms a spherical layer over the cornea. The space between the back of the contact lens and the front surface of the cornea, which is filled with the eye's natural tear film, can counteract an irregular cornea surface.

The soft disposable contact lens is the most popular lens available because of its level of comfort and ease of use. Note the soft center of the lens.

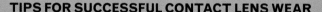

TIPS FOR SUCCESSFUL CONTACT LENS WEAR

- After inserting your contact lenses, rinse the case with warm water and allow it to air dry thoroughly. Cases should be cleaned or replaced regularly.
- Use commercial, rather than homemade, cleaning solutions. Homemade cleaning solutions have been linked to eye infections and may cause discomfort.
- Do not sterilize contact lenses that are designed to be discarded after use.
- Do not mix different brands of solutions.
- Wash your hands with soap prior to handling your contact lenses or touching your eye.
- Do not share your contact lenses with another person.
- Only use fashion color lenses that have been fitted by an eye doctor.
- Do not buy bootleg contact lenses.
- Wear your contact lenses on a schedule prescribed by your eye doctor.
- Do not put your contact lens in your mouth and then in your eye.
- Call your eye doctor if you notice any unusual symptoms and do not wear your contact lenses until your eyes have been thoroughly checked.

Toric lenses are available if you have moderate astigmatism. Toric lenses are shaped with two curvatures so they can correct your specific case of astigmatism and move less when you blink because of their design.

Multifocal contact lenses are an option if you are presbyopic and need help with reading but would rather avoid reading glasses. These are available in soft disposable materials or rigid gas permeable forms. There are several designs available, but all basically combine distance and near correction in a single contact lens.

While it may be tempting to wear your contact lenses longer than prescribed, it is best to adhere to the manufacturer's recommendations to make sure that your eyes stay comfortable and to lessen your risk of eye infections and contact lens allergies.

Monovision lenses are an alternative for presbyopia. In this scenario, your dominant eye is corrected for distance vision while your non-dominant eye is corrected for near vision, each using a single vision contact lens. The quality of the vision tends to be slightly better with single vision contact lenses compared to multifocal contact lenses, but your depth perception may be slightly diminished.

Other types of contact lenses

Although less well-known than the previously mentioned lenses, there are other contact lenses available that have definite benefits.

Rigid gas permeable lenses are not as widely worn as soft disposable lenses, but many people still choose them because they offer several advantages. These lenses are a more modern version of old hard contact lenses and are most often made of silicone acrylate, which is a combination of silicone and a gas-permeable material. They tend to allow a lot of oxygen to permeate the lens and reach your cornea.

Because of their rigidity, however, they aren't always as comfortable as soft disposable contact lenses and it may take you longer to adjust to them. Toric and multifocal contact lenses are available in rigid gas permeable materials. Rigid gas permeable contact lenses are especially useful in correcting irregular astigmatism, so if you have specific corneal problems (such as corneal scars or you have undergone

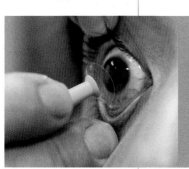

THE RIGHT FIT

Remember that finding the right pair of contact lenses is like finding the right pair of sneakers. Even if you think you know what size you need, you may still need to try several pairs before deciding which pair works best for you.

corneal surgery), you may see better using this type of contact lens rather than glasses.

Hybrid lenses are a combination of soft and rigid gas permeable contact lenses and have recently been gaining in popularity. A hybrid lens has a rigid center but a soft surrounding skirt. It therefore combines the visual advantages of a rigid gas permeable contact lens with the comfort of a soft contact lens. These lenses are also available in multifocal types.

Corneal refractive therapy

If you have mild or moderate nearsightedness or astigmatism and would like to rely less on contact lenses and glasses, you could consider corneal refractive therapy. During this therapy, you wear certain specially fitted rigid gas permeable contact lenses at night, causing a temporary change in your cornea's shape. This change in shape is designed to eliminate your need for contact lenses or glasses during the day. If the lenses are no longer worn at night, the curvature of your cornea will gradually revert to its original shape. This is one of the few instances in which wearing lenses overnight may be advisable, although the risk of eye infections from sleeping in contact lenses is still not zero.

Cosmetic contact lenses

If you've always wanted to change the color of your eyes, cosmetic contact lenses are available in many varieties. Tinted fashion lenses can change the color of your iris, so changing your eye color is as simple as inserting a contact lens. Although these types of color contact lenses do not require a prescription, it is recommended that you consult your eye doctor to have the lenses properly fitted. Other types of cosmetic lenses help you correct or hide eye problems. If your eyes do not have an iris (which can be caused either by injury or genetic defect), you may benefit from cosmetic contact lenses that have a colored iris "painted" on them. Likewise, someone who has had an eye injury can wear a contact lens with an artificial pupil, or someone with a disfigured eye can have a contact lens "painted" to match the iris of the other eye. For complex eye problems, it's important you have a good eye doctor who is experienced in contact lens fitting.

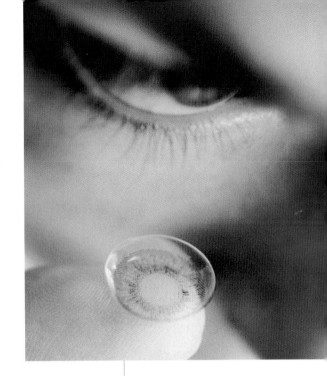

A colored contact lens shows the pattern of the colored iris that has been printed onto the lens.

OPTICAL ILLUSION

With contact lenses widely available for order over the phone and online, many people purchase lenses without consulting an eye doctor. However, having regular check-ups is important and often leads to better results.

Cleaning your lenses

There are two basic methods available for cleaning and disinfecting your contact lenses.

Multipurpose solutions are the most commonly used, primarily because you can clean and disinfect your soft contact lenses using just one solution. Multipurpose solutions are simple and relatively quick, and the cleaning agents in them tend to be mild and well-tolerated, although occasionally they can be irritating to some people.

Hydrogen peroxide involves cleaning your contact lenses and then disinfecting them with a separate hydrogen peroxide solution, which is neutralized during the process. While this method is somewhat cumbersome, because you need separate solutions for cleaning and disinfecting, the lenses tend to be cleaner and there are no preservatives left on them at the end of the process.

Risks of wearing contact lenses

Wearing contact lenses can sometimes cause corneal infections, including corneal ulcers. These infections, while usually treatable with antibiotic eyedrops, can be very serious and can damage your vision long-term by causing corneal scarring or perforation (holes in the cornea). Other complications can include dry eyes and allergic reactions that can cause the conjunctiva, or the outermost covering of the eyeball, to become inflamed (giant papillary conjunctivitis).

The risk of infection increases if you wear lenses while you sleep. You should never wear disposable lenses longer than the recommended timespan. Also, the number of hours a day your eyes can tolerate wearing lenses is limited. See an eye doctor regularly to make sure your contact lenses are not being overworn, which can lead to intolerance and serious corneal problems. It's a good idea to always have a back-up pair of glasses so you can give your eyes a break.

Wearing lenses does not provide protection against eye injury. If you wear lenses while playing sports, for example, you should make sure to follow the recommendations for safety glasses. If you have good vision in only one eye and wear a contact lens in that eye because it corrects your vision better than glasses, you should still wear polycarbonate eyeglasses over the contact lens for best protection.

Refractive surgery

Refractive surgery is available if you want to reduce your reliance on glasses and contact lenses. Surgery that improves your eyes and can treat nearsightedness, farsightedness, and astigmatism has become immensely popular in recent years. The most common type involves an excimer laser, which uses energy in the ultraviolet spectrum of light to reshape your cornea. This type of surgery was pioneered in the early 1960s, but many technological advances have been made since then. As of 2007, over 17 million people worldwide have undergone LASIK surgery, making it one of the most common types of surgery performed today.

Flap procedures

Refractive surgery procedures can be categorized by the technique used. The most common involves a partial-thickness corneal flap, and LASIK (laser assisted in-situ keratomileusis) is the most frequently performed of this group of procedures. The surgeon uses a microkeratome, or blade, to cut a partially hinged flap of corneal tissue typically 100-180 micrometers thick. The flap is lifted, the laser removes tissue from the underlying cornea to reshape it, and then the flap is laid back down. Recently, the IntraLase laser has been developed to cut the flap without using an actual blade, making it more regular in thickness. LASIK is an outpatient surgery using topical anesthesia, or numbing drops.

"Wavefront" LASIK is computer software used during LASIK surgery to achieve more personalized results. "Wavefront" technology attempts to correct tiny aberrations, or irregularities, that may exist in your individual corneal shape. Wavefront technology may result in better refractive results.

Non-flap procedures

In contrast, surface procedures reshape the cornea without creating a flap.

PRK (photorefractive keratectomy): the laser removes the outermost surface of the cornea, changing its shape. This differs from LASIK because

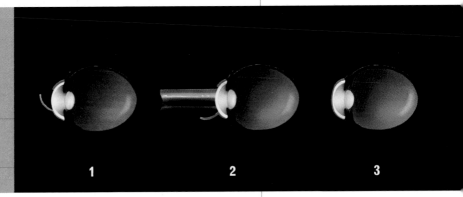

LASIK SURGERY

Nearsightedness can be corrected by flattening a steep cornea.

1 A flap is cut in the cornea using a microkeratome.

2 The laser then removes tissue from the corneal stroma (pink).

3 The flap is then replaced.

no flap is created, so you will have to wear a bandage contact lens while the surface of your cornea heals. Healing time is longer than with LASIK and there may be more discomfort, but PRK reduces the risk of complications from the flap and the final outcomes are similar.

LASEK (laser assisted sub-epithelium keratomileusis) is a combination of the two most commonly performed techniques—LASIK and PRK. To begin, your surgeon uses an alcohol solution to loosen the outermost layer of cells of your cornea, then lifts that 50-micrometer layer with a specialized surgical blade. This layer is thinner than a typical LASIK flap. After your cornea is reshaped by the laser, the outer cell layer is replaced and heals without a visible flap, unlike the corneal flap in LASIK. The discomfort during the healing period is similar to PRK, but the healing time may be shorter.

While the goal of refractive surgery is to reduce your dependence on glasses or contact lenses, you might still need glasses or contact lenses for specific tasks.

EPI-LASIK is a new technique similar to LASEK, except a newer specialized blade is used to lift the top layer of cells, rather than alcohol and the older-style blade. As with LASEK, that top layer of cells is replaced after the laser reshapes the underlying cornea. Avoiding alcohol may make the healing process more comfortable for you.

PRK, LASEK, and EPI-LASIK are all performed under topical anesthesia as an outpatient. If your cornea is too thin to have LASIK performed safely, you may be a good candidate for one of these surface procedures because a permanent corneal flap is not created.

Other refractive surgeries

Although the following types of surgery are not as widely performed as the previously mentioned laser procedures, they are still available. Ask your eye doctor for further details on which procedure would be best for you.

Thermal keratoplasty makes a ring of 8 or 16 burns on your cornea to shrink its tissues and change its shape to correct farsightedness and certain types of astigmatism.

LTK (laser thermal keratoplasty) is similar to TK (keratoplasty) in procedure except, that during LTK, a Holmium laser is used to create the corneal burns.

CK (conductive keratoplasty) is like thermal keratoplasty but uses a high-frequency electric probe to create the burns.

Intacs is the procedure where intrastromal corneal ring segments are implanted in your cornea to correct small amounts of nearsightedness or astigmatism. The Intacs devices are crescent-shaped plastic segments that work by flattening the cornea once they are implanted.

Phakic intraocular lenses act like implantable contact lenses to correct nearsightedness. During surgery, the lens is implanted in front of your eye's natural lens, correcting higher degrees of nearsightedness than laser procedures without depending on your cornea being of a minimum thickness. The lens is also removable if necessary. While having such a lens implanted in your eyeball is slightly more invasive than some other surgeries, it can be a good option.

Cataract surgery is also a type of refractive surgery. After a cataract is surgically removed, the eye surgeon chooses the type and strength of the lens implant. Many of us will undergo cataract surgery during our lifetimes. If you have cataracts that significantly affect your vision, you may benefit more from cataract surgery than from the corneal refractive surgeries mentioned above.

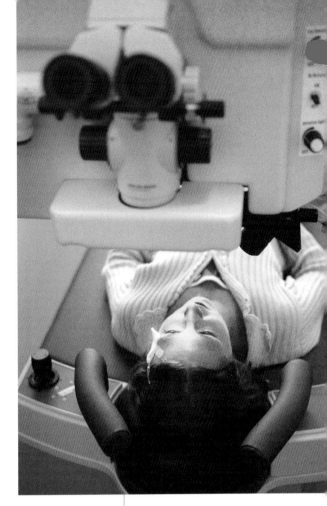

Less common refractive surgeries

Older surgery techniques such as RK and AK have largely been replaced by laser procedures, but are still being performed. Newer techniques, such as transscleral light therapy, are still being tested.

RK (radial keratotomy). The eye surgeon makes radial incisions in your cornea using a diamond blade to correct nearsightedness and/or astigmatism.

AK (arcuate keratotomy). Similar incisions are made at the edge of your cornea to treat astigmatism. AK can be combined with cataract surgery to reduce any astigmatism that is still present after the cataract is removed.

Transscleral light therapy is a new refractive surgery technique that uses a laser to strengthen the ciliary body in order to try to stimulate your eye's ability to accommodate, thus improving your reading vision without the need for reading glasses or contact lenses. This procedure is still experimental and not yet widely available. Further testing will determine whether it is safe and effective.

Refractive surgery is a quick and relatively painless procedure; nevertheless, it has risks you will need to consider.

REFRACTIVE SURGERIES

PROCEDURE	DESCRIPTION	BENEFITS	RISKS
LASIK	A corneal flap is cut; the laser reshapes the cornea underneath the flap; and the flap is replaced.	Most common type of refractive surgery so much experience with this technique; very little discomfort during or after surgery.	Over- and under-correction, dry eyes, glare, halos, infection, inflammation, corneal scarring; thinned cornea may be weaker.
PRK	The laser removes the surface layer and underlying tissue of the cornea to reshape it; the surface layer grows back on its own.	May work better for corneas that are too thin for LASIK or for eyes with large pupils; no corneal weakening since there is no permanent flap.	Over- and under-correction, dry eyes, glare, halos, infection, inflammation, corneal scarring; pain while healing; takes longer to heal than LASIK, LASEK, or epi-LASEK.
LASEK	Alcohol and a blade are used to lift the surface layer of the cornea; the laser reshapes the underlying corneal tissue, and the surface layer is replaced.	May work better for corneas that are too steep or thin for LASIK; no corneal weakening since there is no permanent flap.	Over- and under-correction, dry eyes, glare, halos, infection, inflammation, corneal scarring; pain while healing; takes longer to heal than LASIK; alcohol may be irritating.
EPI-LASEK	A surgical blade is used to lift the surface layer of the cornea; the laser reshapes the underlying corneal tissue; and the surface layer is replaced.	May work better for corneas that are too steep or thin for LASIK; no corneal weakening since there is no permanent flap; avoiding alcohol used in LASEK may be more comfortable and gentler on cornea.	Over- and under-correction, dry eyes, glare, halos, infection, inflammation, corneal scarring; pain while healing; takes longer to heal than LASIK.
RK	Radial cuts are made with a diamond blade in the cornea to reshape it.	Older technique has longer follow-up studies available.	Over- and under-correction, dry eyes, glare, halos, infection, inflammation, corneal scarring; results may change over time; not as common now as other surgeries.
AK	Incisions are made along the edge of the cornea to reduce astigmatism.	Can be combined with other eye surgeries to help correct astigmatism.	Over- and under-correction, dry eyes, glare, halos, infection, inflammation, corneal scarring; may be difficult to predict results.

REFRACTIVE SURGERIES

PROCEDURE	DESCRIPTION	BENEFITS	RISKS
Thermal keratoplasty	A ring of burns is made in the cornea to reshape it.	No corneal weakening since there is no permanent flap.	Over- and under-correction, dry eyes, glare, halos, infection, inflammation, corneal scarring; results may change over time.
LTK	A laser is used to create a ring of burns in the cornea to reshape it.	No corneal weakening. Using a laser may be more precise than thermal or conductive keratoplasty.	Over- and under-correction, dry eyes, glare, halos, decreased contrast sensitivity, infection, inflammation, corneal scarring, results may change over time.
CK	An electric probe is used to create a ring of burns in the cornea to reshape it.	No corneal weakening since there is no permanent flap.	Over- and under-correction, dry eyes, glare, halos, decreased contrast sensitivity, infection, inflammation, corneal scarring; results may change over time.
Intacs	Plastic devices are implanted within the cornea to change its shape.	Implants can be removed if necessary; no permanent corneal flap created; may be useful for abnormally steep corneas.	Over- and under-correction, glare, halos, decreased contrast sensitivity, infection, inflammation, corneal scarring; more difficult surgical technique than LASIK.
Phakic intraocular lenses	Plastic lenses are implanted inside the eyeball to correct nearsightedness.	May work better for very nearsighted eyes; no permanent corneal flap created.	Over- and under-correction, glare, halos, infection, inflammation, cataract formation; problems with eye pressure, corneal cloudiness; more invasive than LASIK; newer technique so riskier.
Cataract	The eye's natural lens is removed and replaced with an artificial lens implant to change the eye's refraction.	Most common type of refractive surgery performed; improves best potential vision by removing blurriness from the cataract.	Over- and under-correction, bleeding, infection, inflammation, retinal detachment, double vision, loss of vision, after-cataract; more invasive than LASIK.

Risks of refractive surgery

While refractive surgery is successful in most cases, it is "real surgery" and has risks and potential complications, just like any other type of surgery. You need to have realistic expectations of the procedure, healing process, and results. With LASIK, 90 percent of patients achieve vision of 20/40 or better without glasses or contact lenses, and 65 percent achieve 20/20 or better. Approximately 3 percent of refractive surgery patients experience a complication within six months after surgery; most are mild, but 0.5 percent are considered serious and require further treatment or maintenance.

The most common complication is over- or under-correction, which can be fixed. Dry eyes may also feel drier, particularly since your eyes are healing. Glare, halos, or minor reductions in contrast sensitivity are a problem for some people. Severe complications, such as eye infections, corneal scarring, or cells growing abnormally underneath the corneal flap, are possible but rare.

Since most refractive surgeries are designed to correct distance vision, many middle-aged people will need help with reading vision after undergoing refractive surgery. If you are nearsighted and presbyopic and are able to read without glasses or contact lenses before refractive surgery, you may need glasses or contact lenses to help you read after surgery. Certain conditions make refractive surgery unadvisable:

- If you are considering refractive surgery, you should be at least 18 years old, and even at this age you should be aware that the refractive state of the eye may not stabilize until your mid-20s.

A corneal topographer projects bright rings onto the eye. The reflections allow an accurate model to be built of the shape of the cornea.

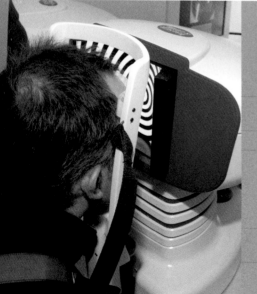

DURING SCREENING FOR REFRACTIVE SURGERY

You should have the opportunity to meet your surgeon at this visit and ask as many questions as needed to make you feel comfortable.

Your vision and need for glasses will be checked.

Your eye pressure will be measured, and a microscope will be used to look at the front part of your eyes.

Your eyes will be dilated to look at your optic nerves and retinas.

Your cornea will be scanned to look for astigmatism and any other irregularities, and your corneal thickness will be measured. These corneal measurements may be used to program the excimer laser, which uses this information as the basis for sculpting your cornea during surgery.

Your pupil size will be measured, and your eyes will be assessed for dryness.

The movement of your eyes should be checked to rule out misalignment.

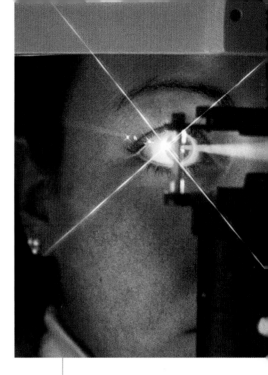

- If you are pregnant or have glaucoma, certain corneal or retinal problems, a history of uveitis (inflammation of the inside of the eyeball), diabetes, vascular disease, autoimmune disease, or problems with wound healing, you may not be a good candidate.
- If you have had ocular herpes within the last year, you should not have surgery performed.
- Certain types of extreme nearsightedness, farsightedness, or irregular astigmatism may not be suitable. It's important to have a surgeon who will perform a full eye examination prior to surgery.

Because refractive surgery usually works by thinning the cornea and a corneal flap is not as strong as the original cornea, an eye that has undergone refractive surgery may be more prone to damage if injured. For this reason, if you play contact sports or activities, you should take special care to wear protective eyewear after surgery.

How to prepare for refractive surgery

Choosing the right surgeon is very important. Some surgeons have had additional specialized training in corneal and refractive surgery, although many fine surgeons have not. Make sure you feel comfortable with your surgeon. He or she should be at your initial eye exam before the surgery and available to answer any questions you have. Your surgeon should also be the same practitioner who examines your eyes during post-surgery visits.

The cost of refractive surgery can be considerable. It is usually considered an elective surgery, so medical insurance often does not cover it as a benefit. Be sure to get upfront and in writing all costs that will be associated with the surgery and then have a plan for meeting them. It is also important that your expectations for the results be realistic. Surgery does not necessarily guarantee freedom from glasses or contacts. While the goal of surgery is to reduce your dependence on glasses or contact lenses, you might still need glasses or contact lenses for specific tasks. Remember that your eyes continue to change throughout your life and will continue to do so even after surgery.

Prior to your surgery, you should avoid wearing contact lenses. Contact lenses can affect the shape of the cornea, so not using them will give your corneas a chance to adjust back to their regular shapes. Your surgeon will recommend the amount of time you will need for this adjustment.

The day of surgery

On the day of surgery, wash your face with soap and water; do not apply eye makeup. Eating a light meal before surgery is generally allowed, but take care to avoid alcohol or medications that can make you drowsy. You should have

The laser requires less than a minute to sculpt and reshape the tissue of your cornea.

someone drive you to and from the surgery. Just prior to the actual surgery, you will be given anesthetic eyedrops and antibiotic eyedrops. You may be given a light sedative, but you will be awake for the procedure.

It is common, although not necessary, for both of your eyes to have refractive surgery on the same day. The surgery generally takes about 10–15 minutes per eye. Most people don't feel any pain, but experiencing some pressure during the surgery is common.

When your surgeon is finished with the procedure, you may be given eye shields or protective glasses to wear overnight. You should relax for the rest of the day. Some people notice irritation or the feeling that "something is in the eye" after surgery; this is common and should gradually fade.

Step-by-step LASIK

During LASIK surgery, the patient lies on a reclining chair or bed. The surgical eye is draped and given numbing eyedrops, and the surgeon marks the cornea with ink to guide future placement of the corneal flap.

An eyelid holder is placed to keep the eye open, and a suction ring is placed on the cornea to pressurize and stabilize the eye; your vision will dim while the ring is in place. A corneal flap is then created, using either a microkeratome blade or a laser. The suction ring is removed and the surgeon gently folds back the flap, exposing the underlying corneal tissue.

The excimer laser is positioned over the cornea and sculpts the corneal tissue while the patient focuses on a fixation light; this part of the surgery generally takes less than 60 seconds. The surgeon will then replace the corneal flap and smooth its edges; he or she may wait several minutes to ensure that the flap remains bonded in place. A protective eye shield may be placed over the surgical eye.

After surgery

You will most likely be checked by your surgeon the day following the surgery and then periodically thereafter, depending on how your eyes heal. You may be given a prescription for eyedrops to use, if your surgeon recommends them. You will probably notice a change in your vision the day after surgery, though it takes up to several months to heal fully. Many people are able to drive the day after surgery, but you should check with your doctor. Your doctor may also recommend avoiding strenuous activity for several days or weeks after surgery. For at least a week after surgery, refrain from using eye makeup to reduce the risk of infection. You should also avoid getting soap or water in your eyes. Swimming should be avoided for up to several weeks. If you have questions about specific activities, be sure to ask your surgeon.

REFRACTIVE SURGERY CHECKLIST

ARE YOU A GOOD CANDIDATE?

☐ **Career impact** Does your job allow refractive surgery?

☐ **Medical conditions** Do you have an autoimmune disease or other major illness?

☐ **Eye conditions** Do you have any problems with your eyes other than needing glasses or contacts?

☐ **Medications** Do you take steroids or other drugs that might prevent healing?

☐ **Stable refraction** Has your prescription changed in the last year?

☐ **Pupil size** Are your pupils extra large in dim conditions?

☐ **Corneal thickness** Do you have thin corneas?

☐ **High or low refractive error** Do you use glasses or contacts only some of the time? Do you need an unusually strong prescription?

☐ **Tear production** Do you have dry eyes?

☐ **Cost** Can you really afford this procedure?

RISKS AND LIMITATIONS

☐ **Overtreatment or undertreatment** Are you willing to have more than one surgery to get the desired result?

☐ **May still need reading glasses** Do you have presbyopia?

☐ **Results may not be lasting** Do you realize that long-term results are not known?

☐ **May permanently lose vision** Do you know some patients may lose some vision or experience blindness?

☐ **Dry eyes** Do you know that dry eyes could worsen, or you may develop chronic dry eyes?

☐ **Development of visual symptoms** Do you know about glare, halos, and that night driving might be difficult?

☐ **Contrast sensitivity** Do you know your vision could be greatly reduced in dim light?

☐ **Bilateral treatment** Do you know the additional risks of having both eyes treated at the same time?

☐ **Patient information** Have you read the information booklet about the laser being used for your procedure?

HOW TO FIND THE RIGHT DOCTOR

☐ **Experience** How many eyes has your doctor performed refractive surgery on?

☐ **Equipment** Does your doctor use an FDA-approved laser for the procedure you need? Does your doctor use each blade only once?

☐ **Long-term care** Does your doctor encourage follow-up and management of you as a patient? Your pre-op and post-op care may be provided by a doctor other than the surgeon.

☐ **Be comfortable** Do you feel you know your doctor and are comfortable with an equal exchange of information?

☐ **Informative** Is your doctor willing to spend the time to answer all your questions?

PREOPERATIVE, OPERATIVE, AND POSTOPERATIVE EXPECTATIONS

☐ **No contact lenses prior to evaluation and surgery** Can you go for an extended period of time without wearing contact lenses?

☐ **Take a few days to recover** Can you take time off to rest for a couple of days if necessary?

☐ **Expect not to see clearly for a few days** Do you know you will not see clearly immediately?

☐ **Be prepared to wear an eye shield** Do you know you need to protect the eye after surgery to avoid injury?

☐ **Read the informed consent** Has your doctor given you an informed consent form?

☐ **Be prepared to take drops** Are you willing to put drops in your eyes at regular intervals?

☐ **Expect some pain/ discomfort** Do you know how much pain to expect?

Courtesy of U.S. FDA

3

Eye Afflictions

Many eye problems are so common that you have probably experienced at least one of those described in this chapter. While reading this book isn't a substitute for going to see your eye doctor, understanding these common problems can help you ask informed questions at your eye appointments and give you insight into the type of problem you or someone you know may have.

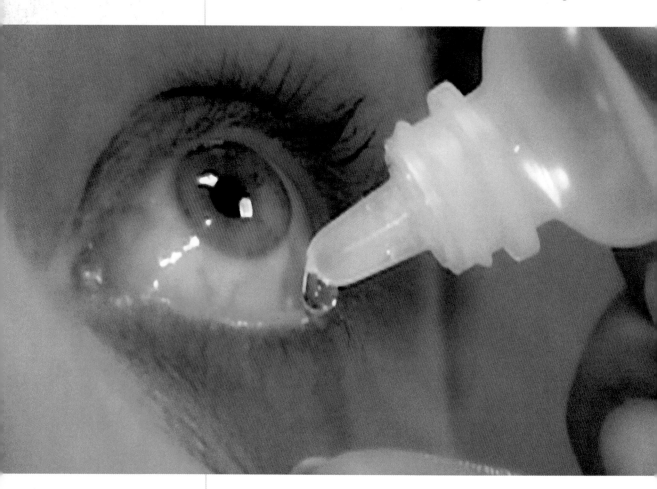

The red eye

Nearly everyone has experienced a red eye at some point in their lives. Many things can cause your eye to turn red, some of which are not harmful, while others can be more dangerous. Understanding what may be causing your eye redness may help you manage your particular situation.

Subconjunctival hemorrhage

If you've ever noticed a bright red patch on the white part of your eye, this is usually due to bleeding from one of the tiny blood vessels under the conjunctiva, or outermost layer of tissue over the white part of the eyeball. This bleeding can happen in almost anyone with no obvious cause, or it can be linked to coughing or straining, using blood-thinning medications, or an eye injury. Less commonly, high blood pressure or a bleeding disorder can be the cause of subconjunctival hemorrhages, particularly if they occur often.

This type of bleeding by itself isn't dangerous for your eye; it usually goes away on its own in 1–2 weeks. Typically, you won't experience a change in vision or pain with this problem, except for perhaps a little mild irritation. If you do notice mild irritation from this spot of redness, you can try using over-the-counter artificial teardrops several times per day for relief.

In the rare case that another medical problem, such as uncontrolled high blood pressure or a bleeding disorder, is causing subconjunctival hemorrhages, your eye doctor may refer you to your family physician for further treatment.

Episcleritis

Episcleritis means inflammation of the episcleral vessels, or blood vessels on the surface of the eyeball beneath the conjunctiva, or outermost layer. It may look similar to scleritis (see page 52). It most commonly causes redness in one area of the white part of your eye, and while the area may be tender and sore, typically your vision remains normal. You should see an eye doctor for this problem so that more serious problems can be discounted.

SUBCONJUNCTIVAL HEMORRHAGE

See an eye doctor promptly if you notice a subconjunctival hemorrhage and:

- You have experienced a recent eye injury.
- Your vision is blurry.
- You have significant eye pain.
- You have double vision.
- Your eyeball is bulging forward.
- The spot of bleeding happens frequently or does not go away after several weeks.

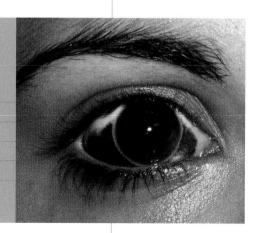

Although episcleritis generally has no known cause, your eye doctor will look for signs of infection or any other medical problems you may have. If the inflammation is very mild, your eye doctor may treat you with artificial teardrops for lubrication. If the inflammation is more severe, she may prescribe a mild steroid eyedrop or an oral anti-inflammatory medicine. Typically, episcleritis goes away, although it can recur.

Scleritis

Scleritis is the inflammation of the deeper blood vessels within the sclera, or thick white wall of the eyeball. It is a more dangerous cause of eye redness but, fortunately, it's less common than episcleritis. The eye pain it can cause is usually more severe than it is in episcleritis, and your vision will usually be blurry. If you notice these symptoms, see an eye doctor promptly, as this disease can worsen and lead to dangerous thinning of the wall of the eyeball. Fifty percent of people with scleritis will have an associated connective tissue disease, such as rheumatoid arthritis or systemic lupus erythematosus or, less commonly, a widespread infection. Your eye doctor may recommend blood tests to look for these illnesses if you have scleritis. She will also examine your eyes thoroughly, since scleritis can cause inflammation in many parts of the eyeball, not just in the front part where the redness is visible. Once an infection is ruled out with laboratory testing, the treatment for scleritis usually starts with oral anti-inflammatory medicines. If these medicines do not control your disease well enough, you may be given oral steroid medicines. Finally, your doctor can consider other immunosuppressive medications if these types of medicines fail or cause problematic side effects.

Conjunctivitis

Almost everyone suffers from "pink eye" at some point in their lives. Conjunctivitis is inflammation of the conjunctiva (the outermost layer of the eyeball) and is one of the most common reasons to have a sore eye. Conjunctivitis can occur for several reasons, such as viral infection, bacterial infection, allergies, or as a side effect of eyedrops.

If you have conjunctivitis, you may notice that the white part of your eyeball is pink or red. There may be discharge, matting of your eyelashes, and a feeling of irritation in your eye. The condition may start in one eye and then spread to your other eye. You might also notice that someone else at home or around you has the same "pink eye," since this problem can be very contagious.

IF YOU HAVE VIRAL CONJUNCTIVITIS:
- Avoid touching your eyes.
- Avoid touching other people.
- Avoid sharing towels and linens.
- Wash your hands frequently.
- Handle and clean all eyewear properly.

Viral conjunctivitis is the most common culprit when it comes to conjunctivitis.

This type of viral infection, like the common cold, usually improves on its own over several weeks. When a virus is responsible for "pink eye," your eye may itch, the discharge from your eye is typically watery, your vision is normal or close to normal, and you may have had a recent head cold. Your eye doctor will be able to distinguish viral "pink eye" from other causes of conjunctivitis when she examines your eyes. She may recommend over-the-counter artificial teardrops and cool compresses for comfort. Rarely, a virus can cause cloudy spots in the cornea, which is then treated with mild steroid eyedrops. Viral conjunctivitis is very contagious for the first 10–12 days, so be careful to avoid touching your eyes and then touching other people or things.

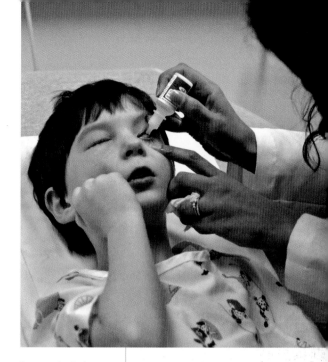

An ophthalmologist treating a young boy with bacterial conjunctivitis.

Herpes simplex conjunctivitis is also caused by a virus, but is slightly different than typical viral "pink eye." Herpes simplex virus usually causes more pain and burning than other types of viral conjunctivitis. Your eye doctor may see characteristic signs of this type of viral infection when examining your eyes, such as blisters on your conjunctiva or eyelids. If you have this type of conjunctivitis, your eye doctor will probably prescribe specific anti-herpes medicines for you.

Bacterial conjunctivitis can be a more serious problem than typical viral conjunctivitis. When "pink eye" is caused by bacteria, your eye will tend to have a puslike discharge, but itching usually isn't as troublesome. While many types of bacteria can cause conjunctivitis, the bacteria that cause gonorrhea are the most dangerous because they can invade the eye quickly and aggressively. Fortunately the gonorrhea-causing bacteria are fairly rare. If your conjunctivitis appears to be bacterial and is severe, your eye doctor may take swabs of your conjunctiva for culture to identify the bacteria causing the problem. The recommended treatment for bacterial pink eye is antibiotic eyedrops, except in the case of gonorrheal conjunctivitis, which is also treated with systemic antibiotics (given by mouth or as an injection into a muscle).

OPTICAL ILLUSION

While many people believe the herpes simplex virus that causes most eye problems is very contagious, this virus lives in our environment and over 90 percent of adults have been exposed to it. Most of us won't ever have an eye problem because of it, even though it's all around us.

Allergic conjunctivitis is related to allergies including hayfever. If you have a history of such allergies and you notice that your eyes are often red, watery, and itchy, then you may be suffering from allergic conjunctivitis.

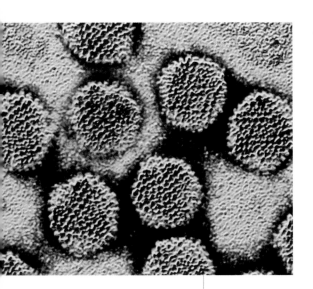

An electron micrograph of adenovirus particles that are associated with eye infections, such as conjunctivitis.

Your eye doctor may be able to distinguish this type of allergy from other causes of conjunctivitis when she examines your eyes. The best treatment for this problem is to eliminate whatever is causing your allergy as much as possible. Also, if your conjunctivitis is mild, over-the-counter artificial teardrops several times a day can help. For moderate allergic conjunctivitis, there are over-the-counter as well as prescription antihistamine eyedrops that relieve the itching, redness, and watering. In severe cases, your eye doctor may prescribe mild steroid eyedrops for a short time. Also, taking antihistamine medications by mouth may help the allergies that affect the rest of your body as well as your eyes.

Eyedrop conjunctivitis may occur if you use medicated eyedrops regularly. Medicated eyedrops can sometimes cause your eyes to become red. Sometimes the preservatives in the drops are the culprit since everyone has a different level of sensitivity to them, while at other times, the medication is causing the irritation and redness. Not using the eyedrops that are responsible (after consulting your eye doctor) is usually the best thing to do in this situation.

Other eye infections

Infections can affect other parts of your eye besides the conjunctiva and still cause red eye. They are primarily spread by respiratory droplets, or particles left on towels and faucets. Good hygiene, including thorough hand washing, is an important way on lessening the chance of infection.

Infectious keratitis is the term for infection of the cornea, or the clear central "window" of your eyeball. These infections are usually caused by bacteria, although fungal infections, herpes virus, or noninfectious causes can all cause similar looking problems. If you sleep with your contact lenses in or don't clean them properly, you will be at higher risk of developing infectious keratitis.

Sleeping with your contact lenses in can increase your risk of developing a corneal infection or infectious keratitis.

If you have this type of corneal infection, you might notice red eye, eye pain, light sensitivity, discharge, decreased vision, or new difficulty wearing your contact lens. You should see your eye doctor promptly for these problems, since diagnosing and treating this type of infection early can make all the difference. Your eye doctor will probably treat you with antibiotic eyedrops, and it may take several weeks for the infection to clear up. If you wear contact lenses, or if the infection doesn't improve, your eye doctor may take swabs of your contact lens or contact lens case or scrapings from your cornea to identify the bacteria that is causing the problem. Stop wearing your contact lenses while the infection is present, and don't resume contact lens use until your eye doctor gives you permission to do so.

Endophthalmitis is an infection that affects the entire inside of your eyeball. Usually, this severe infection either follows an injury that penetrates the eyeball or, in rare cases, can occur after eye surgery. In very ill people, bacteria and fungi in the bloodstream can occasionally settle in the eye, also causing this type of eye infection. Endophthalmitis leads to a red eye with severe pain and loss of vision. If you notice these symptoms, particularly after an eye injury or eye surgery, see an eye doctor immediately as endophthalmitis is an emergency.

SEE AN EYE DOCTOR IMMEDIATELY...

if you experience a red eye with severe pain or loss of vision, especially after an eye injury or following eye surgery.

The treatment of endophthalmitis depends on how advanced it is. For most cases, an injection of very potent antibiotics into the eyeball is the first line of treatment. Your eye doctor may take cultures of the fluid inside the eye to try to identify the bacteria causing the infection. Certain advanced cases may benefit from surgery to clear out the infection from the back part of the eyeball as well as antibiotics administered to the inside of the eyeball. After these interventions, your eye doctor will probably prescribe strong antibiotic eyedrops. Once the infection is controlled, steroid medicines may then be given. Some eyes that have had this type of infection recover and see well, but many others don't return to good vision because the infection and the inflammation it causes can seriously damage the inside of the eye.

Cellulitis

While the other infections that are discussed above can cause your eyeball to be red, cellulitis is an infection that causes redness of the eyelids and skin around your eye. Bacteria are almost always responsible for causing cellulitis, and they usually come from a skin injury, an insect bite to your eyelids, or from your sinuses. It is divided into two types, preseptal cellulitis and orbital cellulitis, depending on its location.

Preseptal cellulitis describes infection of the eyelids and skin around your eyeball that doesn't extend into your orbit, or eye socket. You may notice redness, tenderness, and a swelling of your eyelids that can make it hard to open your eye. In some cases, you may also have a mild fever. In preseptal cellulitis, the eyeball itself may be

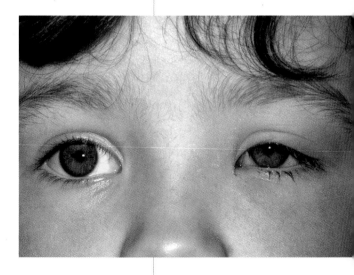

Swollen tissue around the eye of a young girl, caused by orbital cellulitis, a bacterial infection of the skin and its underlying tissues.

slightly red, but is otherwise normal. If you suspect that you have cellulitis, see an eye doctor promptly because, in most cases, this condition needs to be treated with oral antibiotics. If the infection does not improve with oral antibiotics or, if it occurs in a very young child, your doctor may recommend admission to a hospital and a course of intravenous antibiotics.

Orbital cellulitis is much more serious than preseptal cellulitis because the infection is located in the eye socket, closer to the brain. Usually the same bacteria that cause sinusitis can cause orbital cellulitis as well. In these cases, not only will the skin of your eyelid be tender, red, and swollen but your eyeball may also bulge or not move properly, and you may notice pain with eye movements. If you have these symptoms, see your eye doctor immediately. After examining your eyes, she may order an imaging scan of your eye sockets and sinuses if she suspects that you have orbital cellulitis. She may also order blood tests to look for infection. Typically, people with orbital cellulitis are admitted to a hospital and given intravenous antibiotics. If an abscess develops in the eye socket, it may need to be drained surgically.

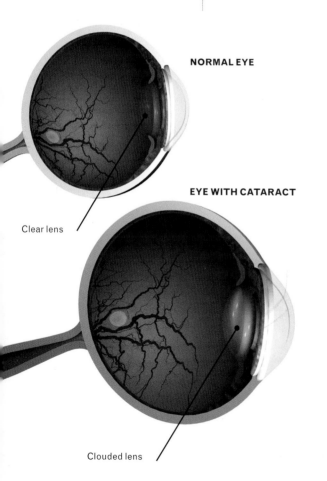

NORMAL EYE

EYE WITH CATARACT

Clear lens

Clouded lens

Cataracts

Most of us know someone who has a cataract or has had cataract surgery. A cataract occurs when the lens inside the eye, which is naturally clear when you are born, becomes cloudy. While aging is the most common reason for someone to develop a cataract, this condition can also be caused by eye injury, using steroids or certain other medications, radiation exposure, diabetes mellitus, inflammation in the eye, and other eye diseases. Smoking and ultraviolet-light exposure can make cataracts worse. Occasionally babies are also born with cataracts.

Symptoms of cataract

Cataracts usually develop slowly over years so, if you have a cataract, you may notice that your vision is gradually becoming blurry over time in one or both eyes. Glare from bright lights, particularly at night, may be problematic. Colors may seem duller and more muted as well. A cataract can gradually cause your glasses prescription to change, typically making you more nearsighted than you were before the cataract developed.

Diagnosing and treating cataract

Your eye doctor can see whether or not you have cataracts when he examines your eyes. If your cataracts are mild, no treatment is necessary. However, if your cataracts are cloudy enough to significantly affect your vision and your ability to perform the activities that are important to you, it may be time for you to consider cataract surgery. Some people may benefit from cataract surgery to make it easier for their eye doctors to follow another eye problem they have, such as macular degeneration (see page 60) or diabetic retinopathy (see page 87), even if the cataract is not directly affecting their vision. If you and your eye doctor decide you could benefit from cataract surgery, she will perform a thorough eye exam with your eyes dilated to determine the overall health of your eyes and measure for a lens implant (see page 58).

Cataract surgery

Nearly all of us will develop cataracts if we live long enough. Over 1.5 million cataract surgeries are performed each year in North America, for example, and many developed countries have similar rates of cataract surgery. The surgery is usually performed on an outpatient basis, and many people have surgery under local anesthesia with mild sedation.

Cataract surgery involves taking out the cataract lens either by using an ultrasound machine to break the lens up and remove its pieces through a tiny incision in the eyeball, or by removing the lens intact through a larger incision. Then a plastic lens implant is placed inside your eye and remains there indefinitely. The entire procedure typically takes less than one hour. If both your eyes have significant cataracts, your surgeries will be performed one eye at a time, usually at least several weeks apart.

On the day of surgery wash your face with soap and water and avoid wearing eye makeup. Don't eat or drink anything starting at midnight of the night before surgery, or according to your surgeon's recommendation. Bring a list of all your medicines with you to surgery, and arrange for someone to drive you to and from the surgery. Depending on the type of anesthesia you receive, you may be awake or asleep for the procedure. If you are awake, you may see some bright lights and feel some eye pressure during the surgery.

After your cataract surgery, your eye may be dressed with an eye shield. You should plan to relax for the rest of the day. Some people notice irritation or the feeling that "something is in the eye" following the surgery, but don't worry—this is normal. Your surgeon will give you instructions about when to start the eyedrops they prescribe for you after your surgery.

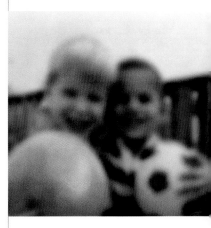

A scene as it would appear to a patient with cataracts. A cataract causes the patient's sight to become blurred and yellowed, and if left untreated, will obscure the vision completely.

Once you've developed a significant cataract, the only effective treatment is to remove the cataract with surgery.

After surgery your eye surgeon will, most likely, check you the day after your operation and then periodically thereafter, depending how you heal. He will give you a prescription for eyedrops to use as your eye heals. These drops typically include an antibiotic eyedrop to prevent infection (some surgeons will ask you to start an antibiotic eyedrop before surgery), a steroid eyedrop to control inflammation, and, in some cases, a second anti-inflammatory eyedrop. You should avoid strenuous activity for 1 week or longer after surgery, upon the recommendation of your surgeon. Some eye doctors will ask you to wear eye protection for part or all of the healing period. If you have questions about specific activities that you may wish to do after surgery, be sure to ask your surgeon.

It typically takes 4–8 weeks for your eye to heal fully after cataract surgery, depending on the size of the incision created during the operation. When your eye is healed, you'll be checked to see if your eye needs glasses, and you may be ready to have cataract surgery for your other eye if it also has a significant cataract.

OPTICAL ILLUSION

While it's tempting to believe that antioxidant vitamins help prevent cataract formation, studies have yet to find any definite benefit from them.

Risks of cataract surgery are low and usually outweighed by its benefits. Ninety-five percent of cataract surgeries go well, but it's important to remember that any surgery involves the risk of complications. With cataract surgery, in particular, there are risks of bleeding, infection, inflammation, problems with eye pressure, retinal detachment, double vision, unintended refractive result, and loss of vision. In some cases, months or years after a cataract extraction, an after-cataract may develop, and your eye doctor will have to examine it (see page 60). Be sure to take the time to talk to your surgeon and understand these risks and your individual potential benefit when deciding whether or not cataract surgery is right for you.

A lens implant can be placed during cataract surgery to also correct any refractive error you may have. Your lens implant will determine whether or not you will need glasses after cataract surgery and, if you do, what your glasses prescription will be. Most people who are undergoing cataract surgery will choose to have a lens implant to correct their distance vision and will typically still need reading glasses afterward. If you wish to be glasses-free after surgery for both distance and near vision, there are relatively new multifocal lens implants available that help reduce the need for glasses for distance and near vision. These multifocal lens implants cost more than single-vision lens implants and have varying degrees of success. If you're interested in this option, discuss it with your surgeon prior to cataract surgery.

QUESTIONS TO ASK YOUR EYE DOCTOR

- **What are my options when choosing my lens implant for cataract surgery?**

- **Am I likely to need glasses for distance or near vision after my cataract surgery?**

Another alternative to reading glasses after cataract surgery is to implant monovision lens implants. This means that one eye will have a lens implant placed to correct distance vision, while your other eye will have a lens implant that corrects near vision. This solution tends to work especially well if you have worn monovision contact lenses successfully in the past.

If you have astigmatism and are about to undergo cataract surgery, typically your astigmatism will still persist after the surgery and may require correction afterward. There are options available to try to reduce the amount of astigmatism that you may have. One option is to implant a toric implant that is designed to correct the astigmatism; another option is to perform arcuate keratotomy, or AK (see page 43), at the time of surgery to reduce your astigmatism.

It's important to remember that aiming for a particular refractive result does not guarantee that you won't need glasses at all after cataract surgery. While the instruments that measure your eye to determine the correct strength of lens implant have made major strides in recent years, these measurements may not be absolutely perfect. If you undergo refractive surgery prior to cataract surgery, for example, it may be difficult to measure for a lens implant. Also people who are nearsighted or farsighted and have a significant cataract in only one eye, may not be able to avoid glasses for the eye with a cataract after surgery, because doing so would create too much imbalance with their other eye. The best, and most realistic, way to think of your refractive result after cataract surgery is as a reduction in your reliance on glasses, not a definite guarantee that you will not need them.

A surgeon performs a cataract extraction on a patient's eye using phacoemulsification.

TIPS FOR MAKING YOUR CATARACT SURGERY A SUCCESS

- **Feel comfortable with your eye surgeon; have a chance to meet and talk to her prior to surgery.**

- **Understand the benefits and risks that apply to your particular cataract situation.**

- **Remember that in general, the time to have cataract surgery is when your cataract bothers your vision enough so that the benefits of surgery outweigh its risks.**

- **Discuss your refractive goals with your surgeon prior to surgery.**

- **Tell your surgeon prior to surgery if you take any blood thinning medications, such as aspirin or warfarin, or prostate medications such as tamsulosin (Flomax).**

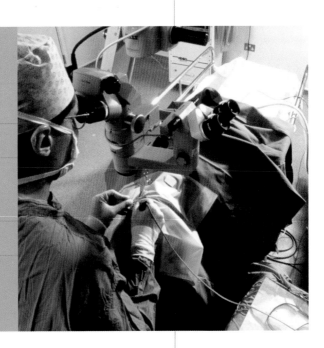

After-cataract

Some people who have had cataract surgery may feel at some point that their cataract has come back because their vision gradually becomes blurry again. This can be due to "after-cataract," which is a film that can form behind your lens implant at any point after cataract surgery. This film (also known as posterior capsule opacification) occurs in up to 25 percent of people in the years following cataract surgery and can cause vision to become blurry again. The reason it can develop is that traces of microscopic cells from the cataract are often left behind, since it's nearly impossible to remove every single cell during the surgery. These cells may grow over your eye's natural support structure, which holds your lens implant in place, forming a film behind the implant that can blur your vision. If you develop such a film, you may notice a gradual blurring of the vision and glare with bright lights, much like the symptoms of your original cataract.

If your after-cataract film affects your vision significantly, your eye doctor can perform a laser procedure to remove this film in her office. This laser is an outpatient procedure usually performed using numbing eyedrops for anesthesia. The risks associated with this laser are small, but include: retinal detachment, high eye pressure, shifting of the lens implant, and swelling in the retina or cornea. Once the film is removed, it usually doesn't recur.

Macular degeneration

When you hear the term "macular degeneration," you may automatically assume it's a severe, blinding disease in all cases. However, in reality, macular degeneration has a broad spectrum, from very mild cases that hardly affect vision at all to severe cases that cause a large central blind spot.

Macular degeneration tends to affect older adults. The disease also tends to run in families, and recent research has begun to identify some genes that are responsible, at least in part, for developing macular degeneration. Other factors that may raise your risk for developing macular degeneration include being Caucasian, smoking, having high blood pressure and/or heart disease, being exposed to ultraviolet light, and eating a fatty diet.

OPTICAL ILLUSION

While "macular degeneration" sounds scary to many people, this disease fortunately doesn't affect the entire retina, so it can't cause total blindness by itself. Most people who suffer from it, even those severely affected, maintain vision that still allows them to get around on their own.

Symptoms of macular degeneration

If you have macular degeneration, you may notice blurry vision in one or both eyes, which comes on either gradually or suddenly. Other hallmarks of the disease include distortion of your central vision, causing straight lines to look wavy, for instance, and central blind spots. These blind spots can make it difficult or impossible to read or to recognize faces. Colors may also

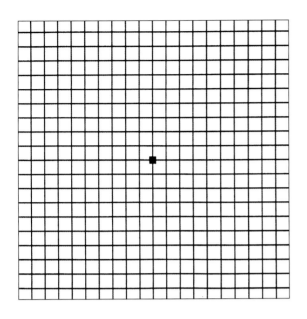

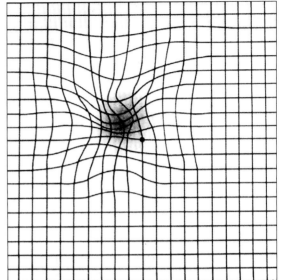

become harder to distinguish. If you have macular degeneration, using an Amsler grid (above) at home can help you monitor any distortion in your central vision.

Dry versus wet macular degeneration

Macular degeneration can be divided into two categories: the dry form and the wet form. Both types start with aging deposits of abnormal material underneath the retina called drusen. These deposits can be linked to damage of the support cells underneath the retina, whose job it is to keep the retina healthy. This relatively early stage is considered the dry form of macular degeneration and, if mild, your vision may still be quite good. The dry form can lead to serious vision loss if the cells under the retina are severely affected in later stages of the disease.

In some cases, macular degeneration can also develop from the dry form into the more advanced wet form if the disease weakens the supporting layer of cells under your retina enough that abnormal blood vessels grow through your retina. These abnormal blood vessels can bleed and leak fluid in your retina, causing even more problems with your central vision.

Diagnosing macular degeneration

When your eye doctor examines your eyes for macular degeneration, she will most likely dilate your eyes to look at your retinas. She will be looking for signs of macular

TOP LEFT Amsler grid representing perfect eyesight.

TOP RIGHT Amsler grid viewed with macular degeneration.

TO USE AN AMSLER GRID

- Keep the grid in a place where you'll see it, and remember to look at it every day or two (that is on the refrigerator or by your bathroom mirror).

- Cover one eye so you test the other eye by itself.

- Stare at the central dot on the grid pattern with one eye at a time; you're looking for new distortion or new blind spots in the grid that you didn't notice before.

- If you notice new distortion or a new blind spot, see your eye doctor promptly.

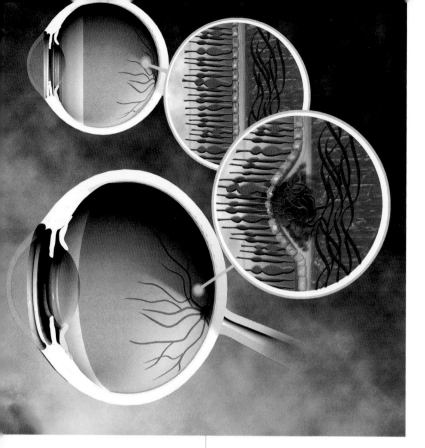

degeneration in your central retina, or macula, such as drusen; abnormalities in the cells underneath the retina; and any signs of bleeding or leaking fluid in the retina. You may have specialized photographs taken of your eye to help evaluate these problems; some of these photographs involve dye being injected through a vein in your arm to better visualize the blood vessels in your retina that may be involved in the disease.

Treating macular degeneration

If your eye doctor diagnoses the dry form of macular degeneration, there's no specific treatment that can improve this condition. Fortunately, many cases of dry macular degeneration don't cause severe vision loss. A recent large study by the United States National Institutes of Health called the Age-Related Eye Disease Study (AREDS) found that certain high-dose antioxidant vitamins can reduce the risk of the dry form of macular degeneration progressing to the wet form by 25 percent. Another recent study by the National Eye Institute suggested that lutein and zeaxanthin (nutrients found in eggs and green vegetables) may also be protective in macular degeneration. If you have macular degeneration, speak to your eye doctor to see if she recommends these vitamins for you.

A healthy eye (top) and an eye affected by wet age-related macular degeneration (bottom). Details of the back of the retina are shown in the circles at the right. The photoreceptors (red and green) are shown with the blood vessels that supply the eye behind them.

AREDS ANTIOXIDANT VITAMINS FOR MACULAR DEGENERATION:

- The recommended daily dosage is: 500 milligrams of vitamin C, 400 international units of vitamin E, 15 milligrams of beta-carotene, 80 milligrams of zinc, and 2 milligrams of copper.

- Numerous formulations of this vitamin combination are available in pharmacies, so read the labels carefully to make sure that you're getting the recommended vitamins and dosages.

- Beta-carotene at this high dosage may increase the risk of lung cancer in current and former smokers, so if you smoke or have smoked, speak to your eye doctor about your need to avoid beta-carotene.

- Inform your doctor if you decide to take these high-dose vitamins.

Treatment of wet macular degeneration has made enormous progress in recent years. Most severe vision loss from macular degeneration is due to the wet type, so having better treatments for this has the potential to substantially improve the lives of many affected people. In the past, the bleeding and leakage from the abnormal blood vessels in wet macular degeneration were treated with different types of laser to preserve the vision from deteriorating further, but vision rarely improved. Now new medicines have been developed to slow down and stop these problematic abnormal blood vessels, and not only are they quite effective in doing so, but in many cases, your vision can even improve after treatment. These medicines are called anti-angiogenic or anti-Vascular Endothelial Growth Factor drugs, and the two most commonly used are Avastin and Lucentis (available in Ontario and Quebec in Canada). These medicines are injected into the eyeball, and the injections are typically repeated every 1–2 months until the disease stabilizes. While injections into the eyeball can be painful and carry small risks of infection, bleeding, and retinal detachment, the benefits often counteract these risks.

While research continues to make great strides in treatments for macular degeneration, living with some degree of vision loss can be an unfortunate reality for whom it affects. Seeing a low vision specialist who can help you maximize your remaining vision and finding out about resources for the visually handicapped in your community may help you to make the most of your vision so you can enjoy the highest quality of life possible (see "Living with Visual Impairment" on page 76).

TEST YOUR
Eye Q:
True or False?
Having a close relative with glaucoma makes you 4–9 times more likely to develop the disease.

True

Macular degeneration affects 30 percent of people aged 75–85 in the United States, over 800,000 Canadians over the age of 40, and many more millions of people throughout the world.

Glaucoma

Does someone you know have glaucoma? This is the second most common cause of blindness worldwide and tends to occur most frequently in advanced age, although occasionally it also occurs in children and babies.

Glaucoma affects your optic nerve, the nerve that carries visual information from your eye to your brain so that you can see. It is made up of approximately one million nerve fibers, and some of these fibers naturally tend to die slowly over time. In glaucoma, the fibers die faster than usual and, if enough of them are lost, your vision can suffer. In the most common form of glaucoma (open-angle glaucoma), damage to your vision tends to progress very slowly over years and can "sneak up" on you before you even realize your vision is no longer normal. It's a good idea to see an eye doctor regularly so the disease can be caught and treated early if it occurs.

Glaucoma tends to run in families, although many people have it without having a known family history. Researchers have discovered several genes that are linked to glaucoma, although much remains to be learned about its causes. Other risk factors for glaucoma include advanced age, being of African or Hispanic descent, having high eye pressure (the pressure inside your eyeball), having thin corneas, migraines, and possibly nearsightedness and high blood pressure.

Open-angle glaucoma

In open-angle glaucoma, the most common form of glaucoma in North America, deterioration of the optic nerve can occur before you even realize it's happening. It's estimated that a person can lose up to half the nerve fibers in their optic nerve from glaucoma before their vision is affected. When vision changes do occur, your side vision tends to be damaged first. A person can have severe side vision loss without noticing it in day-to-day activities. If glaucoma isn't treated and the disease is very aggressive, the central vision can be diminished or lost, sometimes resulting in blindness. In general, glaucoma damage can't be undone once it has occured.

Angle-closure glaucoma

Angle-closure glaucoma is a serious and often sudden condition that occurs when the internal drainage area, or angle, of your eyeball is closed preventing the fluid that fills your eyeball (aqueous humor) from draining out properly from your eye. If this drainage angle closes suddenly and completely, your eye pressure can become dangerously high very quickly. This sudden angle-closure glaucoma is an eye emergency and can lead to severe vision loss in a matter of hours if not treated, due to the very high eye pressure. If you notice the symptoms of angle closure, go to your nearest emergency room, or see an eye doctor immediately.

Angle closure can also occur slowly over time, rather than suddenly. This slow, insidious, chronic angle-closure glaucoma damages your optic nerve when the drainage angle of your eye is partially closed, causing your eye pressure to

This diagram presents a cross-section of a human eye affected by glaucoma. The arrows represent increased internal pressure.

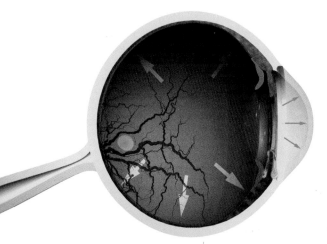

SYMPTOMS OF A SUDDEN ANGLE-CLOSURE GLAUCOMA ATTACK:

- New decrease in vision
- Severe eye pain, possibly with headache
- New halos around lights
- Eye redness
- Nausea or vomiting

be somewhat higher than normal. In this type of glaucoma, the drainage angle does not close off completely and suddenly, as it does in a sudden angle-closure attack. Therefore, your eye pressure typically doesn't climb as high, and you may not experience the severe symptoms of a sudden angle-closure attack. Much like the more common open-angle type of glaucoma, this chronic angle-closure glaucoma can sneak up on you and damage your vision over time without you being aware of the problem.

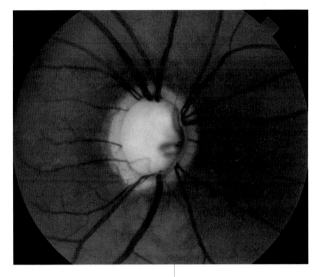

Other types of glaucoma

Other types of glaucoma are less common, but include glaucoma caused by other eye problems, such as inflammation, injuries, genetic diseases, diabetic retinopathy, and blood vessel blockages. The factor that all types of glaucoma have in common is that they all end up damaging your optic nerve.

An image of the retina in a case of glaucoma, showing cupping of the optic disc, a vertical enlargement of the yellow circular area.

Diagnosing glaucoma

When your eye doctor examines you for the possibility of glaucoma, she will pay special attention to your eye pressure and how your optic nerves look. She may use a special lens to examine the drainage angle of each eye. If your doctor suspects glaucoma, she may have you take a special peripheral vision test, designed to look for glaucoma damage to your side vision. In some cases she may order specialized photographs of your optic nerves that search further for glaucoma damage. Since there's no single test that determines whether you have glaucoma, your doctor will interpret your test results collectively and decide if it is likely that you have this disease and whether or not you should be treated for it.

The primary treatment for glaucoma involves lowering your eye pressure to prevent further damage to your optic nerve.

Treating glaucoma

If your doctor decides that you're a "glaucoma suspect" but that you don't have definite glaucoma based on your eye exam, you may just need to be followed regularly in case glaucoma develops in the future.

Open-angle glaucoma is often treated by lowering eye pressure. Even for people who don't demonstrate high eye pressure during a doctor's visit, research has shown that lowering eye pressure can slow down or stop glaucoma from getting worse. Damage from glaucoma isn't reversible, but the goal of treatment is to preserve your remaining vision as much as possible. While there are probably other factors that play a role in causing or making glaucoma worse, such as blood flow to your optic nerve, these aren't treatable at this time.

Lowering your eye pressure can usually be accomplished in three different ways: using pressure-lowering eyedrops regularly, having laser surgery performed in your doctor's office, or having eye surgery in an operating room. Your doctor will discuss these options with you to determine which is best for you. Depending on how severe your glaucoma is, you may need one or more of these types of treatments, and because glaucoma is treatable but not curable, your glaucoma will need to be monitored over your lifetime.

If you have angle-closure glaucoma or drainage angles that are narrow and may therefore be prone to developing angle-closure problems in the future, your eye doctor may recommend a laser treatment designed to open your drainage angles as much as possible. The laser is performed in your eye doctor's office and works by making a tiny hole in your iris (the colored part of your eye). If the laser treatment solves your drainage angle problem, you may just need to have regular eye exams in the future to make sure that glaucoma doesn't develop later on. If you have glaucoma damage already and your eye pressure remains too high even after the laser treatment, you may need to use pressure-lowering eyedrops long-term, or in some cases, have eye surgery in an operating room to better control your glaucoma.

Other types of glaucoma that are linked to other eye problems are often treated by controlling the underlying eye problem. Often, pressure-lowering eyedrops are used to lower your eye pressure, much as in the more common types of glaucoma. In some cases, laser treatments and glaucoma surgery in an operating room can be used to manage these types of glaucoma as well.

With early detection and proper treatment, glaucoma is a manageable condition for most of the people that have it, and it rarely ends up causing blindness. The key is diagnosing the disease early and keeping up with treatments for it in order to best preserve your vision for the rest of your life.

In the United States, over two million people and almost 2 percent of people over age 40 have glaucoma, while at least 300,000 Canadians are affected by it. By 2020, it's estimated that nearly 80 million people worldwide will have glaucoma.

Retinal detachment

Until the last few decades, retinal detachment was a blinding condition that couldn't be treated. Fortunately, medical science has made tremendous progress more recently, and now there are modern surgical techniques that can repair over 95 percent of retinal detachments to attempt to preserve and improve your vision.

Usually, a retinal detachment occurs because a tear or a hole forms in your retina. The aqueous humor, fluid that normally fills your eyeball, can then pass through the tear or hole and get underneath the retina, causing it to detach from the wall of your eyeball much like peeling wallpaper. In the area where the retina is detached from its underlying supporting tissues, vision is lost. Although retinal detachments only occur in 10–15 out of 100,000 people, if untreated, they commonly cause severe vision loss and blindness.

Certain factors make your risk of developing a retinal detachment higher:

Having had a retinal detachment in one eye increases the risk of having one in your other eye by 10 percent.

- People who are nearsighted are more prone to developing retinal tears and detachments. If you're very nearsighted, your risk of having a retinal detachment is up to 10 times higher than that of a person who is not nearsighted.
- Another retinal condition, lattice degeneration, which causes weakening of the peripheral retina, makes you more prone to developing retinal holes that can lead to retinal detachment. Lattice degeneration is present in 6–8 percent of the population, which means that most people with lattice degeneration will never have a retinal detachment.
- If you've had cataract surgery, your overall risk of retinal detachment in the years following surgery is about 1 percent. Having laser surgery for an after-cataract film also has a very small risk of retinal detachment.

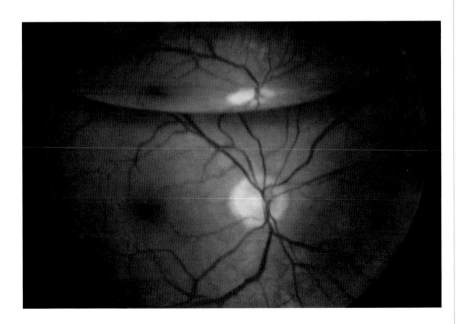

A gas bubble has been placed in this eye to repair a retinal detachment.

- An injury to your eyeball also makes your risk of retinal detachment higher, and these detachments can occur soon after or even years after the original injury.
- Having had a retinal detachment in one eye increases the risk that your other eye will also suffer a retinal detachment at some point.

The risk of retinal detachment is highest in the first several weeks after a posterior vitreous detachment occurs. If you have a newly diagnosed posterior vitreous detachment, be aware of the symptoms of retinal detachment, and see your eye doctor if you experience any of them.

Posterior vitreous detachment

Have you ever noticed floaters in your vision? These floaters are usually caused by a posterior vitreous detachment, which is when the vitreous, or gel, that fills the back part of your eyeball becomes more liquid over time. This gel normally attaches to your retina at certain points. When the gel liquefies, it moves around inside your eyeball, and the gel's attachments pull away from your retina. If the attachments tug hard enough at the retina while separating, your retina can tear. Posterior vitreous detachment happens in most people as they get older, although many don't notice it, and fortunately most of the time the retina doesn't tear. If the posterior vitreous detachment causes new symptoms that you do notice, your risk of retinal tear and detachment is higher than if you didn't notice any symptoms.

Diagnosing retinal tears and detachments

If you have symptoms that are suspicious for a retinal tear or detachment, your eye doctor will dilate and examine your eyes, paying careful attention to your retinas to see if these problems are visible. If she doesn't see a tear or detachment, she may ask you to come back for a follow-up examination a few weeks later in case a retinal tear develops during that time.

SYMPTOMS OF RETINAL TEAR OR DETACHMENT

If you notice the following symptoms, see an eye doctor immediately.

- New floaters
- New flashes of light
- New decrease in vision
- A dark curtain that comes across all or part of your vision

Treating retinal tears and detachments

If your eye doctor notices a retinal detachment, you'll most likely need urgent laser surgery to repair it or stop it from getting worse. Some retinal tears also need this type of treatment, while other types of retinal tears can be watched without treatment to see if they stay stable.

If your retinal tear or detachment is small but needs treatment, your eye doctor may be able to treat it with laser in her office. The laser limits the area of the retina around the tear or detachment to stop it from spreading to other parts of your retina. These treatments work well in most cases, although some people will need to have further surgery if the laser can't stop the tear or detachment from progressing. Your eye doctor can also treat some retinal detachments in her office with an injection of air or special gas into your eyeball to push on the area of detached retina and encourage it to adhere to its proper location. For other larger or more vision-threatening types of retinal detachments, surgery in the operating room may be your best option.

Traditionally, there are two main types of surgery for retinal detachments, and they are sometimes combined:

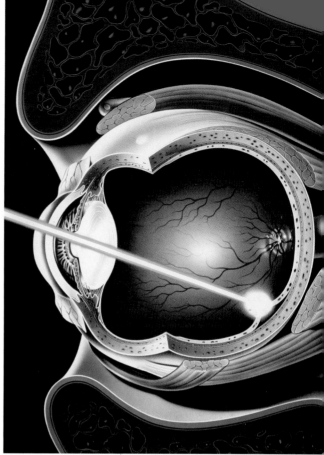

- A band of plastic, called a scleral buckle, can be placed around your eyeball to indent it so that the detached retina adheres to the wall of your eye. This is often combined with laser treatments and gas injected into your eye to help the formerly detached retina stay in its proper position.
- The other method, called vitrectomy, uses tiny instruments to enter the vitreous cavity, or back part of the eye, to remove your vitreous gel and reposition the detached retina from the inside of the eyeball. This too may also be combined with laser treatments and gas injections during your vitrectomy surgery to help repair your retina.

This diagram shows laser surgery on a detached retina. The laser (white) is operating at a point where the retina (yellow) has separated from the choroid.

Based on your type of retinal detachment, your eye doctor will recommend the best method to treat you. No treatment is risk-free, and surgery for retinal tears or detachments carry the risks of bleeding, infection, inflammation, trouble with eye pressure, cataract formation, changing your need for glasses, losing vision, losing the eye, and needing further treatment if your retinal detachment recurs. But because retinal detachments almost never get better on their own and have the potential to cause blindness in many situations, repairing them is generally your best course of action.

Retinal artery and vein blockages

Just as blood vessels in your heart and your brain can become blocked, causing heart attacks and strokes, blood vessels that feed your retina can also become blocked, leading to "strokes" in your eye. Because these arteries and veins normally supply oxygen and other necessary nutrients to your retina, blockages can damage your retina and, in many cases, cause severe loss of vision.

These blood vessel blockages can be classified into those that affect arteries that bring blood to the retina, and those that affect veins that carry blood away from the retina. The consequences and treatments of these different types of blockage are also different, which is why it's important for your eye doctor to decide which type may be affecting you.

Artery blockages

Artery blockages are usually due to fatty debris that blocks the blood vessel. These artery blockages can be either central or branch. A central retinal artery occlusion happens when the main artery that feeds almost your entire retina becomes blocked, while a branch retinal artery occlusion is a blockage of a smaller branch of that main artery that only feeds a portion of your retina. A central blockage tends to have devastating effects on your vision, since this "stroke" to the entire retina means that it completely lacks blood flow. A branch artery blockage, on the other hand, can barely affect your vision or can be much more serious, depending on which branch is blocked and what part of your retina it normally supplies. If the area of the affected retina is close to your macula (the part of your retina responsible for your central vision), the impact of the "stroke" will probably be worse than if the area is farther away from your macula.

> If you've had a central retinal vein occlusion, the chance of vein occlusion occurring again in the same eye or in your other eye is 10 percent in the first two years after the initial blockage.

Vein blockages

Likewise, when the veins of your retina become blocked, the blockage can be either central or branch. Usually, a clot in the vein causes the blockage. In central retinal vein occlusion, the main vein that drains your retina becomes blocked by a clot. While this can cause blindness in some cases, other people may fare better because their blockage isn't as complete. This is in contrast to a central retinal artery occlusion, where the vision ends up being poor in almost all cases. A clot that forms in a side branch of your central retinal vein is called a branch retinal vein occlusion. Similar to a branch retinal artery occlusion, only part of your retina is affected. Likewise, the damage to your vision depends on which part of your retina is involved and how complete the blockage is.

People who are prone to developing these blood vessel blockages tend to be over the age of 50. Not

RETINAL BLOOD VESSEL BLOCKAGES ARE MORE COMMON IF YOU:

- Have high blood pressure
- Have diabetes
- Have bleeding or clotting problems
- Have vasculitis (inflammation of blood vessels)
- Have an autoimmune disease
- Have had a serious eye injury
- Have glaucoma
- Use oral contraceptives

surprisingly, some of the same risk factors that make a person more likely to have other blood vessel problems, such as heart disease and stroke, are also risk factors for retinal blood vessel blockages. Rarely, temporal arteritis can cause a retinal artery occlusion.

Symptoms of retinal artery or vein blockages

If you have a retinal blood vessel blockage, you'll most likely notice sudden, painless loss of vision in one eye. The degree of your vision loss will depend on what size and type of blood vessel is blocked. Some types of blockages occur more commonly when you wake up in the morning. If you notice sudden vision loss, be sure to see an eye doctor right away.

Diagnosing retinal artery or vein blockages

If your eye doctor suspects a retinal blood vessel blockage, he'll likely dilate your eyes to examine your retinas carefully. He'll look for signs such as poor blood flow to your retina or leaking and bleeding from damaged blood vessels that may indicate this type of problem. He may obtain specialized photographs of your retina, some of which may require an injection of dye into a vein in your arm while the photographs are being taken. He may also check your blood pressure and order some blood tests to look for any causes of the blood vessel blockage, or refer you to your primary care doctor for this type of testing.

Treating retinal artery or vein blockages

If you see your eye doctor immediately after a retinal artery blockage occurs, she may try to lower your eye pressure by massaging your eye, using pressure-lowering eyedrops, or withdrawing some of the aqueous humor, or fluid inside the front part of your eyeball, with a tiny needle. Although this only rarely brings back the lost vision, usually the vision loss is severe enough to warrant trying these treatments in case they help at all. After you have a retinal vein or artery blockage, depending on how severe the blockage is, you may need to follow up monthly with your eye doctor for the first few months. Then your visits may be spaced further apart. At these visits, your eye doctor will look for signs of abnormal blood vessels that may grow in your eye as a result of the poor blood flow. These abnormal blood vessels can leak, bleed,

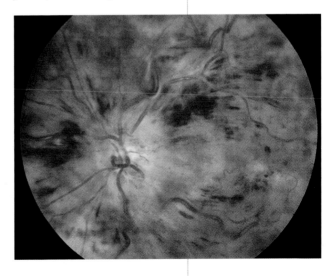

Retinal vein occlusion is the blockage of one or more blood vessels of the retina; in this case, the central retinal vein is blocked, which causes bleeding within the retina.

and cause glaucoma or retinal detachment. If they develop, your eye doctor may recommend laser treatments to shrink them. Some branch retinal vein occlusions in particular can cause swelling in your central retina that can also be helped by laser treatments. For some people, steroid medicines or anti-Vascular Endothelial Growth Factor drugs such as Avastin and Lucentis (also used to treat wet macular degeneration) can be injected into the eyeball to help treat the complications of retinal artery and vein blockages.

> If you've had a retinal vein or artery blockage, it's important to follow up regularly with your eye doctor. Promptly treating any resulting complications can help preserve your eyesight.

Unfortunately, these blood vessel blockages can occur again in your other eye in the future. Controlling glaucoma, if you have it, can help lower the chance that a vein occlusion can happen again. To maximize your chances of avoiding retinal blood vessel blockages in the first place and to reduce the risk of recurrence, remember to take care of yourself and control any high blood pressure, diabetes, and cholesterol problems that you may have. Besides receiving regular eye care, keeping yourself as healthy as possible is the best way to preserve your vision and keep you seeing your best.

Double vision can be monocular (in one eye) or binocular (in both eyes). The medical name for double vision is Diplopia.

Double vision

Double vision will strike many of us at some point in our lives. Double vision occurs when one object looks like two images, or when two images of the same object overlap. Deciding whether the double vision is occurring in just one eye, or in both eyes together, is the most important way to figure out which of many possible causes is responsible for the problem.

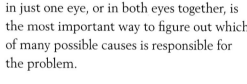

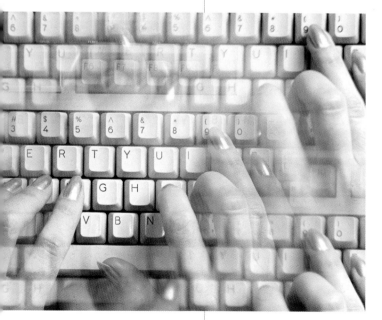

Monocular double vision

If your double vision is just in one eye, meaning that closing the other eye does not make it go away, then the cause is a refractive problem in that one eye itself. This means that for some reason, light entering your eye doesn't focus properly on your retina to form a single image. Dry eye syndrome, a scar or other irregularity in your cornea, or cataract are the most common causes of this type of double vision. Less commonly, a dislocated lens or lens implant after cataract surgery, an irregular iris (such as after eye surgery or an eye injury), retinal disease, or retinal detachment can also cause this problem. Treating this type of double vision depends on its cause.

Binocular double vision

In contrast, if your double vision is present with both eyes open but then goes away when you close one or the other eye, this is a different type of problem called binocular double vision. In this type of double vision, the alignment of your eyes is faulty. In normal situations, your brain compiles the images that each eye sends to it and comes up with a three-dimensional image that you see based on minor differences between each eye's view. If your eyes aren't properly aligned, then your brain receives information from each eye that it can't make sense of to create a single image and, because of this confusion, the resulting image appears double rather than single.

When children have crossed eyes, they usually don't see double because their brains can suppress the image in one of their eyes, allowing them to see a single image. These children tend to have poor depth perception as a result, since seeing an object in three dimensions depends on the brain taking notice of the images coming from both eyes. When adults develop eye misalignment, however, they are much more likely than children to notice double vision because their brains aren't able to suppress one of the images.

Convergence insufficiency may be to blame if you tend to notice double vision that occurs with eye strain and headaches after you've been reading for a while. Normally, your brain causes both eyes to cross inward just slightly to focus on a close object, such as a book. In convergence insufficiency, your brain can't keep your eyes focused together on that close object as you get tired, so you may notice blurry or double vision as a result. Your eye doctor

HOW TO DO PENCIL PUSH-UPS

- Hold out your finger, or a small object such as a pencil, at arm's length and stare at it.
- Keep staring at your fingertip, or the object, while slowly moving it to the tip of your nose.
- Make note of the point where the image becomes double, then hold the object just slightly farther than that point and stare at it for ten seconds.
- Repeat these steps 10 times, 2–4 times per day until you can bring the object all the way to the tip of your nose without it appearing double.

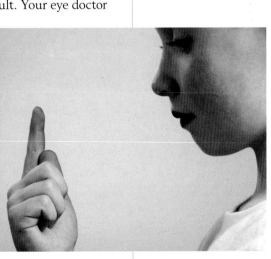

will be able to tell if this is the cause of your double vision by listening to your history and by testing your eye alignment. Convergence insufficiency is one of the only types of eye misalignment that can be treated with exercises. Pencil push-ups (see previous page) or computer programs that exercise the eye muscles responsible for seeing up close can help your symptoms. Alternatively, wearing glasses for reading that have a prism in them can also relieve this type of double vision.

OPTICAL ILLUSION

Babies with severely crossed eyes sometimes alternate which eye they are fixating with to supply the brain with its image. This alternate fixation is protective against developing a lazy eye, since each eye in turn is being used at least some of the time.

Other causes of binocular double vision are drinking alcohol, head injury, certain neurological diseases, and certain drugs and medicines that can affect your brain. If you notice new binocular double vision, see a doctor immediately as this can also be one of the symptoms of stroke. Another cause of this type of double vision is poor function of one of the nerves that controls the eye muscles that move your eyeball. Problems in the part of your brain that controls eye movement can also lead to double vision. Your eye doctor will examine your eyes looking for causes of your double vision and, if necessary, will order testing that will help determine the cause of the problem.

Treatment for binocular double vision depends on whether or not it is persistent. For some people, a prism that bends light to compensate for eye misalignment can be added to their glasses to relieve their double vision. For others, eye muscle surgery to realign their eyes can help. Some people may benefit from injections of botulinum toxin (Botox) into one of their eye muscles to improve their eye alignment. While double vision can be a frustrating problem, most people do well with treatment.

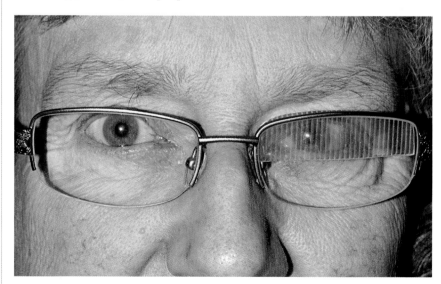

A woman wearing glasses fitted with a temporary adhesive prism to correct double vision.

Lazy eye

Lazy eye, or amblyopia, occurs when your eye doesn't see as well as it should because its connections to the brain didn't develop adequately in childhood. This happens when the eye isn't used fully in childhood, and proper brain connections don't form.

Children whose eyes are crossed or misaligned may develop a lazy eye in one or both eyes. Typically, one eye will become stronger, while the other weaker eye can become useless as the brain directs energy to forming visual connections with only the stronger eye. Children with eye diseases (for instance, children born with cataracts) can develop a lazy eye in an eye that doesn't see well. Other children who need glasses from an early age can develop a lazy eye if they don't wear glasses that allow their eyes to focus properly.

Symptoms of a lazy eye

If you notice that your child has crossed eyes or doesn't seem to see as well as you think she should, take her to see an eye doctor. Also, if you notice that your child's pupil (the black circle in the center of the colored iris) looks whitish instead of black, tell your pediatrician or eye doctor right away as this may be a sign of cataract or rare eye tumor. Because you probably spend more time with your child than anyone else does, you're the person most likely to notice any problems with her eyes. If you do notice something unusual, you should bring it to your family doctor's attention in case it turns out to be a serious problem.

Treating a lazy eye

Detecting and treating a lazy eye early in childhood can make the difference between allowing a child to grow up with an eye that sees well and contributes to good depth perception, and having her live with vision that does not develop properly. The earlier treatment begins, the better. Treatment can range from wearing glasses to correct any nearsightedness, farsightedness, or astigmatism, to eye-muscle surgery to correct crossed eyes or eye misalignment. Many children with a lazy eye wear a patch for a prescribed length of time (up to several hours per day) over their stronger eye to force their other lazy eye to work harder. Similarly, other children use dilating drops in their stronger eye to blur it, which also encourages their lazy eye to develop its visual potential.

While treating a lazy eye works best if it begins at a very young age,

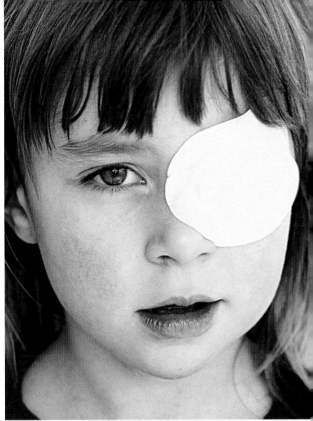

Lazy eye treatment can involve forcing the bad eye to function properly by covering the good eye.

The earlier treatment of a lazy eye begins, the more likely it will be successful.

even teenagers with a lazy eye may benefit from patching or drop therapy. Pediatric eye doctors who specialize in this type of problem can help your child maximize their visual potential so that they are prepared to reach their adult years with the best vision possible.

Living with visual impairment

Many of us consider vision to be the most crucial of senses, since it determines how we function in our daily lives to a great degree. When vision is imperfect, your health and well-being can suffer greatly.

With the baby-boomer generation aging, as well as the global population's life expectancy continuing to increase, many of us will have a close friend or family member who will have to learn to live with imperfect vision as he or she gets older. While much of Western medicine is designed to treat disease, even with the best available treatments, not all vision loss can be prevented. The field of low vision has developed to help those of us who have imperfect vision to make best use of the vision that we still have. This field has helped many visually-impaired people, by using specialized visual aids as well as introducing them to community resources, maximize their quality of life.

OPTICAL ILLUSION

You may think that aging in and of itself can make your vision worse, but, in fact, it's not a given that your vision will worsen just because you are getting older. It's the diseases that occur more commonly as we age that can make our vision worse, not aging itself.

What are legal blindness and low vision?

Legal blindness is defined in North America and in many European countries as vision with best-correction (using eyeglasses or contact lenses, if necessary) of 20/200 or worse or side vision limited to 20 degrees or less from center in your better-seeing eye. This means that when wearing glasses or contact lenses, if the best you are able to see from either eye is the 20/200 "big E" on the eye chart, you would meet the criteria for legal blindness. In Australia, a person who is legally blind may have best-corrected vision of 6/60 or worse or side vision of less than 10 degrees from center in the better eye.

Low vision, on the other hand, is defined as vision of 20/70 or worse in the better eye. Low vision isn't poor enough to meet the requirements for legal blindness. People who are legally blind or have low vision often still have some useful vision, and it can be very helpful for them to see a low vision specialist. Specialists can help them to make the most of the vision that still remains and preserve their independence as much as possible.

The level of vision required to legally operate a motor vehicle varies. In the United States, for instance, this varies from one state to another.

Low vision specialists

Low vision specialists are eye care providers who focus on treatment options for less than perfect vision. An exam with a low vision specialist often starts with this specialized eye doctor asking what work, hobbies, or activities are important to you. She may check your eyes to see if glasses would help your vision for distance or near objects. This refractive testing may differ from that performed in a general eye doctor's office in that specialized devices, such as telescopes, might be used to come up with an optimized glasses prescription. Also, your side vision may be tested, and the low vision specialist might pay special attention to how your eyes move, especially when you read. All of this is designed to find out how your vision can be optimized to improve your independence.

Some low vision specialists also work with occupational therapists that are specially trained to help adapt your home and your activities to your level of vision. An occupational therapist who works with low vision clients may come to your home, for example, to point out ways to set up your furniture and belongings so they are easier and safer for you to manage. The therapist may help label and organize objects so you can most easily perform daily tasks. Some occupational therapists also help with mobility training if your level of vision makes it difficult for you to get around easily.

Community resources

In addition to seeing a low-vision specialist, a person with impaired vision may want to investigate resources available in the community. Many low vision specialists and other eye doctors have information about local support groups for people and families of people with limited vision. These days, online support groups can also provide much-needed contact with others who might be suffering from similar eye problems, and these often extensive online networks can help you connect with them all over the world.

Also, most states in the United States have a government agency, often called a Commission for the Blind, that works with people with impaired vision to provide services that can help them function more fully in today's society. These agencies have listings of resources available to people with impaired vision and are great places to start researching your opportunities. These resources can range from educational opportunities for visually impaired people to financial help in certain situations as well. People with low vision in other countries should ask an appropriate governmental authority what community resources are available to them.

Seventeen percent of people over age 65 in North America have low vision or are legally blind.

QUESTION TO ASK YOUR LOW VISION SPECIALIST

Would I benefit from having an occupational therapist come to my home to show me how best to set up and organize my daily routine?

Because reading is such an important part of life, a significant portion of low vision services addresses the reading difficulties faced by those who are visually impaired. Your local library is likely to have large-print books and newspapers, which can help those with relatively mild vision problems. The United States Library of Congress runs the National Library Service, which organizes a network of libraries that mails Braille and audio materials to eligible low-vision borrowers for free.

Braille was much more widely used in the United States several decades ago, and its usage has decreased dramatically since then. Fortunately, with the advent of more user-friendly computer technology for the visually impaired in recent years, there are other good options for those with imperfect vision to keep up with the world around them.

Visual aid devices

Once your low vision eye doctor has examined you, she can recommend treatments to maximize your existing vision. She will be familiar with optical devices that can make reading or performing other visual tasks easier.

As technology advances, more and more user-friendly optical aid devices are coming onto the market. Many of the newer devices use electronics to magnify

TEST YOUR
Eye Q:

True or False?

Legal blindness is vision of 20|200 or worse OR side vision limited to 20 degrees or less from center in the better-seeing eye.

True

WAYS TO HELP PEOPLE WHO ARE VISUALLY IMPAIRED

- To put the person with low vision at ease, identify yourself and anyone else who is with you when you enter the room.
- Don't rearrange a room or the belongings of someone with low vision without letting the person know.
- Arrange good lighting for tasks according to the person's preference.
- Use contrast wherever possible to make tasks easier, such as writing labels with black marker.
- Use texture to help label things; use puffy fabric paint, tape, or nail polish to mark dials, thermostats, or other objects.
- When describing food on a plate, describe its location in clock-hour format; for example, chicken is at 12 o'clock, broccoli is at 4 o'clock, etc.
- When walking, let the person with impaired vision take your elbow; say out loud if there are steps or obstacles approaching.
- Involve the person with visual impairment in helping decide how best to arrange things at home to make tasks easier.

Courtesy of Dr. Donna Wicker

objects to make them easier to see if you have low vision. This list includes some traditional devices that are commonly used, as well as some recently developed devices that are quite sophisticated. No single device will work for everyone, so if you are interested in purchasing any of these, it's best to see a low-vision specialist first to try the device and see if it fits your individual needs, and to avoid wasting money and time on devices that aren't suitable.

LOW-VISION DEVICES

Optical-aid device	Description
Closed-circuit television system	Video camera magnifies text and projects it onto a large screen.
Extra-strong bifocal glasses	The reading part of the lens in the bottom of a pair of glasses. The lens is made stronger than usual, thus acting as a magnifier.
Headworn electronic magnifier	A visor that is worn over the eyes that has a video camera that magnifies distant objects and projects the image to the inside of the goggles.
Large screen or talking glucose meter	Specialized machines that measure blood glucose levels. Can either display the result in large digits or say the result out loud.
Magnifying glass	Hand held or set on a stand, a traditional magnifying glass makes objects appear larger.
Mobile phone organizer	Cell phone with large buttons and voice-activated functions makes calls, has Internet access, and takes notes.
Portable hand-held electronic magnifier	Tiny video camera magnifies text and projects it onto a liquid crystal display screen.
Screen magnifier	A computer software program that magnifies what is on a computer screen.
Screen reader	Computer software reads computer text aloud.
Voice-response computer	A specialized computer that uses voice recognition to allow you to browse the Internet; available in free-standing form or as software that works with your existing computer.
Wearable telescopes	Telescopic lenses are added to a section of the distance lenses on a pair of glasses.

WEBSITE RESOURCES FOR LOW-VISION OPPORTUNITIES

www.aao.org	The American Academy of Ophthalmology sponsors the National Eye Care Project, which is an outreach program that provides medical eye care to people who need access to an ophthalmologist.
www.afb.org	Helen Keller worked with the American Foundation for the Blind for 40 years. This is a nonprofit organization that lists resources for people with impaired vision. Its website also features online communication forums with other people or families of people with decreased vision.
www.lighthouse.org	Lighthouse International is a non-profit organization dedicated to providing low vision services to those with limited vision. The Lighthouse website allows you to download a free web browser tool for visually impaired people. Located in the New York area, Lighthouse International also provides educational opportunities at its facilities.
www.loc.gov/nls	The National Library Service for the Blind and Physically Handicapped is a division of the United States Library of Congress. It organizes a national network of libraries that provides audio and Braille materials to legally blind borrowers by U.S. postal mail.
www.navh.org	The National Association for Visually Handicapped serves those people with some residual vision in particular. It provides large print reading materials and low vision aids, and it has offices in New York and San Francisco that feature visual aids and ergonomic lighting for people with limited vision.
www.preventblindness.org	Prevent Blindness America is a volunteer organization with local chapters in many locations. Its website contains online fact sheets about eye problems, eye safety and health, and living with low vision.
www.visionaware.org	Vision Aware is a website that lists helpful resources for people with limited vision.
www.blindcanadians.ca	The Alliance for Equality of Blind Canadians serves to increase awareness of rights and responsibilities, so blind, deaf-blind, and partially sighted individuals can have equal access to the benefits and opportunities of society.
www.cnib.ca	The Canadian National Institute for the Blind is the primary source of support, information, and most importantly, hope, for all Canadians affected by vision loss.

EYE EMERGENCIES

IF A BLUNT OR SHARP OBJECT CUTS YOUR EYE OR EYELID	• If available, tape a paper cup over your eye to protect it. • Don't flush your eye with water or any other fluid. • Don't try to remove any object stuck in your eye. • Don't eat or drink anything. • Go to your nearest emergency room immediately for medical attention.
IF YOU RECEIVE A BLOW TO YOUR EYE	• Go to your nearest emergency room immediately if you notice pain, decreased vision, or a black eye. • If you are sure that your eyeball isn't injured, but you notice a bruise or swelling on your eyelids or face, use a cold compress without putting pressure on your eyeball. • Even if you think your eyeball is not injured, see an eye doctor within a few days to make sure your eyeball isn't involved.
IF A CHEMICAL SPLASHES YOU IN YOUR EYE	• First rinse your eye with tap water for 15 minutes to flush out the chemical. • If you're wearing a contact lens, don't try to remove it. • Then go to your nearest emergency room immediately.
IF A SPECK LANDS IN YOUR EYE	• Pull your upper eyelid gently away from your eyeball to see if the speck will fall out. • Let your tears try to wash away the speck. • If your eye irritation doesn't go away, see an eye doctor promptly.
SEE AN EYE DOCTOR PROMPTLY IF YOU EXPERIENCE:	• A decrease in your vision. • A new change in your peripheral vision. • Eye pain. • New painful light sensitivity. • Eye redness, especially if you also have eye pain or wear contact lenses. • New discharge from your eye. • New flashers or floaters in your vision. • New double vision. • Growths, swelling, redness, or tenderness of your eyelid.

4

How Your Health Affects Your Eyes

Your eyes are an integral part of your body and can provide a view into how your body works. For instance, your eyes are one of the only places in your body where your blood vessels can be examined without the aid of special imaging technology. Many diseases that affect the rest of your body can also affect how your eyes function. Your overall health has a direct relationship with your eye health.

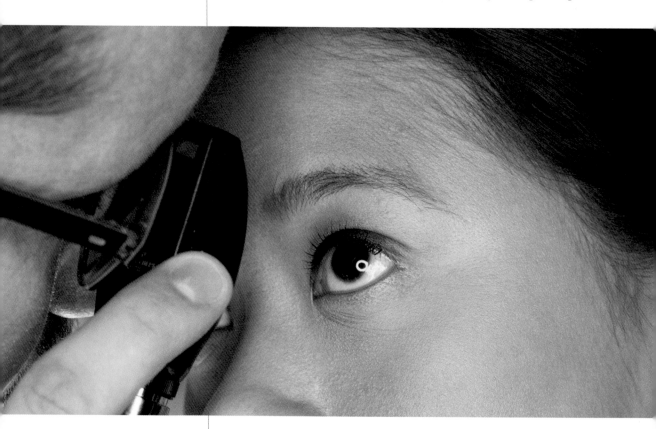

The pathway of your eyes

Did you know that your eyes are physically connected to the rest of your body in several ways? Therefore the health of your body can have an effect on the health of your eyes.

How our eyes connect to our bodies:

- The blood supply to your eyes comes from the ophthalmic artery (a direct branch of the internal carotid artery) that runs through your neck and carries blood from your heart to your head.
- The ophthalmic artery has branches that can be visualized as being divided into two groups: branches that supply blood to your orbit (or eye socket) and branches that supply blood to your eyeball and its muscles. The orbital branches provide oxygen and nutrients to the structures in the orbit, such as the tear gland and orbital fat that supports your eyeball. The branches that supply your eyeball send vital nutrients to each of the six muscles that move your eyeball and then divide into smaller branches that feed the different parts of the eyeball itself.
- The optic nerve is the principal connection between your eyeball and your brain, and it is the "cable" that sends images from your eye so your brain can "see" them. The optic nerve itself can be thought of as an extension of your brain, since like the brain, it's made of nerve cells. The optic nerve is likewise surrounded by a protective coating of tissues that also surround the rest of your brain.
- Several other nerves (cranial nerves) that travel directly from the brain also control your eye's movement and sensation. Some of these cranial nerves carry signals that tell your eye's muscles to contract, which allows your eyes to move together in various directions to look at different things. Other cranial nerves supply your tear glands and eyelid muscles that open and close your eyelids, as well as other muscles in your face.

OPHTHALMIC ARTERY

The ophthalmic artery is a branch of the internal carotid artery that travels from your heart through your neck and up to your brain. The ophthalmic artery itself has many branches that carry blood to your eye and different parts of your orbit. Your eyes rely on this steady blood supply to provide them with the necessary nutrients to function normally.

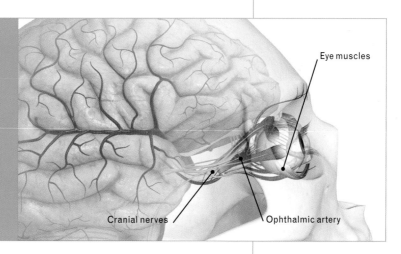

Eye muscles

Cranial nerves

Ophthalmic artery

The fifth cranial nerve in particular sends branches to different parts of your face and eye that relay sensory information back to your brain so you can feel pain, temperature, and touch.

Avoid smoking to keep your eyes healthy

One of the most basic and important things that you can do to maximize the health of your eyes is to avoid smoking tobacco. Besides causing lung cancer and contributing to other diseases elsewhere in the body, smoking is strongly linked to worsening of cataracts, macular degeneration, and thyroid eye disease. Smoking may also be a factor in diabetic retinopathy and glaucoma, although the scientific evidence is still inconclusive for these two diseases. Some researchers have suggested that smoking is linked to anterior ischemic optic neuropathy (or a stroke to the optic nerve), amaurosis fugax (a temporary halt of blood flow to the eye, resulting in a brief blackout of vision), and strabismus (eye crossing or misalignment) in children whose mothers smoked while pregnant. Further research studies are needed to verify these possible relationships.

> Even if you have smoked for a long time, stopping will still have major benefits for your eyes and your health.

Smoking and cataracts

If you smoke, you're up to 2.9 times more likely to develop a nuclear cataract (the most common type of cataract) than someone who doesn't smoke. This risk increases even more with heavy smoking (more than 20 cigarettes per day). Once you quit smoking, your increased risk of developing cataracts begins to lessen over time. It's thought that perhaps the toxins produced from smoking accumulate in the lens of the eye and cause the development of a cataract, or that smoking decreases the level of antioxidants (such as vitamin C) in the lens, that protect against the formation of a cataract.

A cataract is visible as the dense, whitish opacity behind the pupil. Most cataracts occur as people age. Smoking increases the chance of their development by 2.9 times.

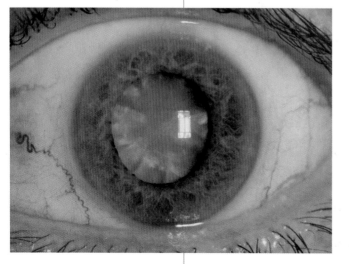

Smoking and macular degeneration

The U.S. Surgeon General has reported that smoking is linked to both the dry and the wet forms of macular degeneration. Studies have shown that the risk of developing any type of macular degeneration is 2–3 times higher in smokers than in nonsmokers, and the risk of developing wet macular degeneration in particular is at least 4 times higher in smokers than in nonsmokers. Once a person quits smoking, his or her risk of developing macular degeneration lessens with time. As with cataracts, the more a person smokes, the higher the risk of developing macular degeneration. The theories behind the association of smoking and macular degeneration suggest that smoking lowers the levels of antioxidants in the bloodstream that protect against macular degeneration, and that smoking reduces the oxygen supply to the retina, which leads to the retinal damage that causes vision loss.

Smoking and thyroid eye disease

Smoking also affects people who suffer from thyroid eye disease. Current smokers are 1.32 times more likely to develop thyroid eye disease than nonsmokers. For light smokers, this risk is slightly less than in heavier smokers. Certain symptoms of thyroid eye disease are particularly sensitive to smoking; for example, the risk of developing double vision from thyroid eye disease is up to 7 times higher in heavy smokers (who smoke more than 20 cigarettes per day) compared to light smokers. As in cataract and macular degeneration, while your genes and other factors in your environment contribute to whether you might develop thyroid eye disease, smoking is the factor you can best control.

Smoking cessation

When it comes to protecting and preserving your own eye health, quitting or avoiding smoking is one of the best things you can do. If you are interested in quitting smoking, the U.S. National Cancer Institute recommends steps to take that will make it easier on you. It is important to set a quit date; tell family, friends, and coworkers about your plans to quit; anticipate the challenges that you'll need to face as you are quitting; and remove tobacco products from your home, car, and workplace.

Your family doctor can give you advice about nicotine replacement products, such as gum, inhalers, lozenges, nasal sprays, and patches as well as anti-depressant medicines that can aid the quitting process. There are community support groups and clinics available to help you stop smoking as well. While we cannot alter our genes or totally control our environment, smoking is a health enemy that we do have the power to stop.

Systemic diseases that can affect your vision

Many diseases that mainly affect the rest of your body can also, unfortunately, have consequences for your eyes and your vision. Some of these diseases are very common, and many of us will encounter at least one of them at some point in our lives. Treating the overall disease is usually the best way to protect your vision and your eye health.

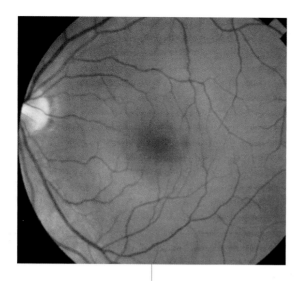

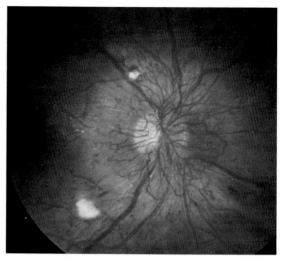

TOP LEFT A fundus photograph (taken with a retinal camera) of a normal retina.

TOP RIGHT A fundus photograph of a retina with diabetic retinopathy.

Diabetes mellitus

Diabetes is quickly becoming one of the most common chronic diseases in the developed world today. In diabetes, your body either does not produce or properly use insulin, which is a hormone made by the pancreas that allows the body's cells to use glucose, a type of sugar. Glucose builds up in the bloodstream and causes damage, both short-term and long-term, throughout the body. Scientists don't fully understand the causes of diabetes yet, but genetics as well as obesity and having an inactive lifestyle may contribute to whether a person gets diabetes.

If you have diabetes, the longer you've suffered from it, the more likely you are to have eye damage from the disease. Diabetic retinopathy is the most common form of eye damage caused by diabetes. In diabetic retinopathy, the blood vessels that supply the retina become damaged from long-standing exposure to high blood sugar levels. These blood vessels can leak and bleed and ultimately become destroyed, which means that the areas of the retina that they should be supplying no longer receive adequate nutrients and oxygen. The blood vessels can also grow abnormally in the later stages of diabetic retinopathy, and these abnormal blood vessels can cause more bleeding, retinal detachment, and neovascular glaucoma, which are serious complications that often lead to severe vision loss.

Diabetes is divided into types 1 and 2:

Type 1 tends to begin in younger people and is characterized by the body's failure to produce any insulin. Therefore, type 1 patients need to take insulin regularly. Type 1 patients are more likely to develop diabetic retinopathy over time than type 2 patients.

Type 2 patients have a resistance to insulin rather than an absolute lack of insulin. Type 2 patients comprise 90–95 percent of all diabetic people in North America, and the incidence of type 2 diabetes is rising quickly in other developed countries. Oral medications, insulin, or a combination of both may be prescribed to treat type 2 patients. Diabetic retinopathy has several stages:

Nonproliferative diabetic retinopathy is its mildest form. The blood vessels throughout your retina start to leak, and tiny spots of bleeding occur. Your vision is usually still normal at this early stage.

It's estimated that 246 million people worldwide have diabetes, and 7 million people develop diabetes each year. By the year 2025, 380 million people are expected to have diabetes.

Diabetic macular edema is swelling caused when blood vessels leak fluid at or near the macula (the part of the retina responsible for central vision) and can occur at any stage of diabetic retinopathy. Diabetic macular edema typically causes vision to be blurry.

Retinal ischemia or lack of oxygen, occurs when diabetic retinopathy progresses. The blood vessels of your retina become damaged and close themselves off. This lack of oxygen tends to make the vision moderately to severely blurry. The bleeding from the damaged blood vessels may also worsen as the disease progresses.

Proliferative diabetic retinopathy can develop in even later stages of the disease. At this stage, abnormal blood vessels grow in an attempt to compensate for the poor function of the original damaged blood vessels. These abnormal blood vessels tend to bleed easily, and they can also scar and contract, which may pull on the retina. Depending on how hard the scar tissue tugs at your retina, it may tear, leading to retinal detachment

CHANCES OF HAVING DIABETIC RETINOPATHY IN TYPE 1 AND TYPE 2 DIABETICS

Risk of diabetic retinopathy	Type 1 diabetics (on insulin)	Type 2 diabetics (on pills, insulin, or both)
After 5 years of having diabetes	25%	40% if on insulin 24% if not on insulin
After 15–20 years of having diabetes	80%	84% if on insulin 53% if not on insulin

and further vision loss. If abnormal blood vessels also grow into the front part of the eye, affecting the iris and drainage angle, the eye pressure may increase because the drainage angle is clogged by the abnormal blood vessels. This is called neovascular glaucoma, which is another vision-threatening problem.

OPTICAL ILLUSION

While many people may think of laser refractive surgery when they hear about laser surgery to treat diabetic eye disease, these treatments use different types of lasers and target different parts of the eye. While refractive surgery lasers can make your vision better, laser treatments for diabetic eye disease generally are designed to preserve your vision, rather than improve it.

Treating diabetes

Mild or moderate nonproliferative diabetic retinopathy doesn't require specific eye treatment beyond regular eye exams and strict blood sugar control, which is the key for all diabetes treatments. If you have severe nonproliferative diabetic retinopathy you may benefit—and with proliferative diabetic retinopathy you will definitely benefit—from laser treatment that reduces your eye's demand for oxygen and discourages the growth of abnormal blood vessels.

Laser treatment can also help diabetic macular edema by clearing up the leaking fluid in your macula. For severe diabetic retinopathy or macular edema that does not respond to laser treatment, newer treatments such as injections of steroid medicines, or anti-growth factor medicines in or around the eyeball can also help to reduce further vision loss. Neovascular glaucoma may require eyedrops and medicines to control eye pressure; in some cases, glaucoma surgery becomes necessary to reduce the pressure.

Ways to reduce the risks of type 2 diabetes

The cause of type 1 diabetes is not known, but there are things that you can do to reduce the risks of developing type 2 diabetes. Maintaining a healthy body weight, avoiding excess sugar in your diet, and exercising regularly can reduce the chance that you may develop diabetes, although there is some genetic predisposition to developing type 2 diabetes that you cannot change. If you already have type 1 or 2 diabetes, preventing blindness from the disease is something that you can control in many cases. It is important to see your eye doctor for regular visits, since studies have shown that receiving timely treatment for diabetic retinopathy can greatly reduce the risk of losing vision. In addition to this, controlling your blood sugar and blood pressure can help slow down the progression of diabetic retinopathy.

One study of type 1 diabetic patients showed that maintaining normal blood sugar levels with insulin resulted in 50–75 percent reductions in diabetic retinopathy development and progression. In the long-term follow-up, the risk of progression was 5 times less with intensive insulin treatment rather than less strict (lax) insulin treatment.

QUESTIONS TO ASK YOUR EYE DOCTOR

- If I have diabetic retinopathy, what stage is it at?

- Do I need laser treatment?

- Is the goal of treating my diabetic retinopathy to stabilize my vision so that it won't get worse, or is there a chance my vision could improve with treatment?

For type 2 patients in another study, intensive (rather than lax), blood sugar therapy resulted in a 29 percent reduction in the need for laser eye treatments. Strictly controlling blood pressure resulted in 34 percent less progression of diabetic retinopathy and 47 percent less vision loss from diabetes.

If you have diabetes, keeping your hemoglobin A1c (a 3-month average of the sugar level in your blood) level as normal as safely possible and controlling your blood pressure are the most important things you can do to preserve your vision and your general health.

High blood pressure

High blood pressure, or hypertension, is extremely common as you get older, and it, too, can have effects on your eyes and your vision. Besides contributing to your risk of stroke, kidney damage, and heart disease, high blood pressure can cause changes in your retina and in its blood vessels. These changes are known as hypertensive retinopathy. Generally the more severe and uncontrolled the high blood pressure is, the greater your risk of developing hypertensive retinopathy.

When an eye doctor examines a person with mild hypertensive retinopathy, she may see narrowing or thickening of the retinal blood vessels. In the mild stages of this disease, vision is not usually affected. In later stages of the disease, there may be bleeding or swelling in your retina because the blood vessels become damaged and leak due to uncontrolled high blood pressure. The optic nerve can become swollen as well. At these later stages, or if blood pressure is extremely high, your vision can become blurry. If the hypertensive retinopathy is very severe, abnormal blood vessels can grow, leak, and bleed just like the abnormal blood vessels that grow in proliferative

EYE EXAM SCHEDULE FOR PATIENTS WITH DIABETES

Diabetes type	Recommended time of first exam	Recommended follow-up*
Type 1	5 years after onset	Yearly
Type 2	At time of diagnosis	Yearly
Type 1 or 2 prior to pregnancy	Prior to conception or early in the 1st trimester	If mild retinopathy or less: every 3–12 months If moderate-severe retinopathy: every 1–3 months

*Your eye doctor will decide if there are abnormalities in your eyes that may make more frequent follow-up visits necessary.

diabetic retinopathy. This can result in retinal complications parallel to those found in severe diabetes.

Besides causing hypertensive retinopathy, high blood pressure can also increase the risk of developing blockages of arteries and veins that supply the retina. These blockages might be thought of as "strokes" to the retina. Such blockages include central retinal artery occlusions, central retinal vein occlusions, branch retinal artery occlusions, and branch retinal vein occlusions. The blockages tend to result in vision loss, depending on the size of the blocked blood vessel, the part of the retina it supplies, and the severity of the blockage. These "strokes" to the retina are usually not reversible.

If you have eye problems caused by high blood pressure, the main treatment is to control your blood pressure as well as possible. One problem with high blood pressure is that it tends to be a silent disease, and you can suffer from it for years without noticing any symptoms. This is why having regular checkups with your primary care physician to screen for high blood pressure is important for good health. If you know that you have high blood pressure, you can best control it by following up regularly with your primary care physician and taking blood pressure medication if necessary. Also watching your diet and getting regular exercise can help keep your blood pressure under control. With hypertensive retinopathy, controlling your blood pressure can help the disease improve and, in some cases, perhaps even help recover some lost vision if the vision loss is due to a short-term rise in blood pressure. However, as a general rule, while eye treatments and eye surgeries can help control some of the complications of hypertensive retinopathy, they generally do not restore lost vision from blood pressure that has been too high for too long. Preventing eye complications from high blood pressure is the key to managing this disease, and the other parts of your body that high blood pressure can damage, such as the brain, heart, and kidneys, will also benefit from good blood pressure control.

> Uncontrolled high blood pressure not only increases the risk of strokes in your brain but also increases the risk of stroke-like blood vessel blockages in the retina.

Blood vessel blockages

Because your eyes, like your other organs, receive their blood supply from your heart, any blockages in the blood vessels that lead from the heart to the eyes can affect how the eyes function. One area where blood flow is especially important is in the internal carotid artery in your neck. This artery carries blood from your heart to your head, and one of its branches is the ophthalmic artery that supplies blood to your eyeball. If the internal carotid artery becomes blocked by atherosclerosis, or hardening of the artery, the eye and the brain may not receive enough blood to function normally.

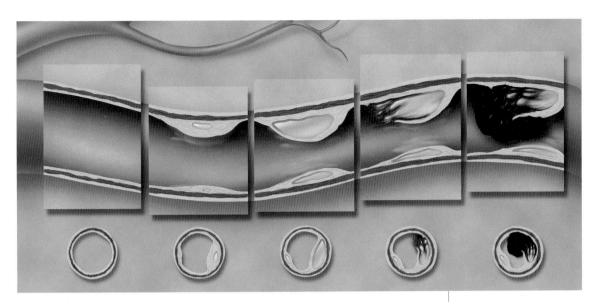

When the eye does not receive enough oxygen and nutrients to function normally, this is called ocular ischemic syndrome. Often this is due to a blockage in the internal carotid artery or in the branch that feeds your eye—the ophthalmic artery. As a result of the poor blood flow, your retina and optic nerve in particular can become damaged, leading to gradual or abrupt vision loss. A cataract can also develop or worsen, and there may be inflammation in the front part of the eye, which can cause eye pain and light sensitivity. Sometimes the eye pressure can be low because the eye does not have enough blood flow to produce its usual amount of aqueous humor, or internal fluid. In the later stages of the disease, abnormal blood vessels can grow as the eye tries to compensate for the lack of oxygen and nutrients. Much like in proliferative diabetic retinopathy, these blood vessels can further damage the retina, grow abnormally in the front part of the eyeball, and cause neovascular glaucoma and dangerously high eye pressure.

The cross section above illustrates the blockage of an artery. The progression of atherosclerosis can lead to the blockage and hardening of the artery, which may prevent the eye and the brain from functioning properly.

The blockages in the internal carotid artery and its branches that cause ocular ischemic syndrome are usually due to cholesterol plaques that line the blood vessels. You may be more likely to develop this problem if you have high blood pressure, diabetes, or heart disease. If you are prone to developing atherosclerosis, this type of blockage can occur in many locations, such as your heart or the blood vessels that supply your legs. Ocular ischemic syndrome tends to happen more commonly in older people, and men are affected more often than women.

IF YOU ARE OVER AGE 60 AND EXPERIENCE VISION LOSS ACCOMPANIED BY:

- **Headache**
- **Jaw pain or fatigue, especially while chewing**
- **Weight loss**
- **Fever**
- **Muscle weakness**

See your eye doctor immediately, since these can be warning signs for temporal arteritis, an eye emergency.

Another uncommon disease that can cause ocular ischemic syndrome is called temporal arteritis. In these cases, poor blood flow to the eye occurs because of inflammation in the arteries that supply the eyeball, rather than cholesterol plaques clogging those arteries. A person with temporal arteritis may have signs of ocular ischemic syndrome in one or both eyes but may also have symptoms such as a headache, jaw pain, weight loss, fever, or muscle weakness. If you are over the age of 60 and you experience such symptoms along with vision loss, you should report them to your eye doctor immediately. If your eye doctor suspects temporal arteritis, she will order lab tests that will check the inflammation levels in your blood or even perform a biopsy to see if there is inflammation in your blood vessels. If she decides you have temporal arteritis, she may recommend treating you with steroid medicines.

If your eye doctor suspects you have ocular ischemic syndrome, she may refer you to your primary doctor for testing to see if there are blockages in the blood vessels in your neck. In some cases, you may undergo an echocardiogram of your heart to see if there are clots being passed from your heart to the blood vessels that supply your eye, causing blockages.

The treatment of ocular ischemic syndrome has two purposes:

- First, your eye doctor will treat any complications or damage to the eye. If your retina has abnormal blood vessels growing and bleeding, those vessels may shrink back and return to normal with laser treatments or injections of medicines into your eyeball. If the eye pressure becomes high, your eye doctor may recommend pressure-lowering eyedrops or glaucoma surgery.

- Second, the underlying cause of the poor blood flow to the eye should be addressed. For instance, if there is severe blockage in the internal carotid artery, some people may benefit from surgery to unblock the artery. For other people, taking blood thinners may reduce the risk of their vision worsening, as well as their risk of stroke or heart disease. Your eye doctor and family doctor will coordinate your care in order to best treat this condition.

OPTICAL ILLUSION

Many people don't realize that a stroke can affect vision, but losing some side vision is a common symptom of a stroke.

Because blockages in the blood vessels that supply your eyes are often linked to blockages in other blood vessels feeding other parts of the body, the risk of stroke and heart disease are higher if you have ocular ischemic syndrome. If you would like to reduce your chances of developing these diseases, it's important to eat a healthy diet, maintain a normal weight, exercise regularly, and avoid smoking. If you have diabetes or high blood pressure, controlling your blood sugar levels and blood pressure will help.

While we can't change our genes, we can try to make our lifestyles as healthy as possible to decrease our risks.

Stroke

When most people think of a stroke, vision loss is not usually one of the first symptoms that springs to mind. But, along with paralysis and difficulty speaking, one common symptom of stroke is losing half of your peripheral vision. A stroke happens when the blood supply to the brain is disrupted for some reason. The most common cause is from a clot that blocks a blood vessel; less commonly, a stroke can be caused by a blood vessel that ruptures and bleeds. Stroke is, unfortunately, a very common disease, and many of us know someone who has suffered a stroke.

When stroke affects the vision, it is usually because the blood supply to the areas of the brain that process visual information has been disrupted. The brain's visual pathway connects the optic nerves, in the front of your head, to the occipital cortex in the back of your head, where brain cells process images so that you can see. Any problems with the brain cells along this long and complex pathway can cause damage to a person's peripheral vision. If the blood supply to the occipital cortex itself is interrupted, vision on either the right or left side, or possibly the central vision, can be lost. The amount of vision loss depends on how large an area of your brain is affected by stroke or how severe the interruption in blood flow is.

Less commonly, stroke can also affect the brain stem from which your 12 cranial nerves originate. Some of these nerves control vision, the muscles that move your eyeball, the muscles of your eyelids and face, and your face's sensation. If these cranial nerves are injured by stroke, one or both eyelids may droop, your eyes may not move together normally, or your pupils may not react normally to light. Most strokes in this part of the brain will also have other serious symptoms besides eye problems, since our brain stems control so many of our body's key functions.

Besides your genes and your age—risk factors for stroke that you can't change—there are several risk factors that you can control:

- The most important risk factor is high blood pressure. A person with uncontrolled high blood pressure has a 35–50 percent higher chance of stroke than a person without high blood pressure. Reducing high blood pressure by even a small amount can greatly reduce your risk of stroke.
- Atrial fibrillation is another important risk factor for stroke. In this condition, the heart muscle quivers instead of beating normally, making the heart prone to developing clots, which can pass to the brain and block its blood supply. As a result, patients with this

TEST YOUR
Eye Q:

True or False?
Untreated atrial fibrillation raises your stroke risk to 5 percent overall.

False
Untreated atrial fibrillation raises your stroke risk to a 5 percent chance of having a stroke each year.

Stroke is the most common cause of disability worldwide.

condition have a 5 percent chance of stroke per year if they are not treated with medications.

- High cholesterol may also be linked to stroke, and the statin drugs used to treat high cholesterol have been shown to lower the chance of stroke by 15 percent.
- People with diabetes are 2–3 times more likely to have a stroke than people without diabetes. This may be partly because people with diabetes also tend to have high blood pressure and high cholesterol.
- Good nutrition may lessen the lifetime risk of stroke according to some studies.
- Avoiding smoking is also crucial.
- For some people with certain risk factors, doctors may recommend low-dose blood thinners, such as aspirin, for stroke prevention.

Eating a Mediterranean diet containing healthy amounts of olive oil and red wine may halve the risk of stroke.

With stroke, 75 percent of people will have significant, lasting deficits from their disease. Because stroke causes so much death and disability, a lot of recent attention has turned to treating stroke as an emergency. If you act quickly when a stroke occurs, this can reduce or even reverse the damage that it causes. If a clot is found to have caused a stroke within three hours of its onset, in some situations, medications can be given to dissolve the clot. This can lead to better outcomes, so it's crucial to go to the emergency room quickly if you notice the symptoms of stroke in yourself or in someone else. These symptoms, besides the vision problems discussed above, include: sudden numbness or weakness, particularly on one side of your face and/ or body; a sudden inability to hear, taste, or swallow, or move the tongue; sudden dizziness or balance problems; new inability to speak or slurred speech; or new difficulty walking or moving. The staff at the emergency room will perform a scan of your brain to determine if a stroke is occurring, and what the cause may be.

Even if clot-dissolving medications are not appropriate treatment for a particular stroke patient, there are other acute treatments that can help. Blood thinners can reduce the risk of further clot formation and worsening or recurrent stroke. Controlling blood pressure appropriately can also limit the damage to your brain. In certain types of strokes caused by bleeding in the brain, neurosurgery may be needed. Also, surgery that unblocks clogged blood vessels in the neck that feed your

WARNING SIGNS OF STROKE—GO TO THE EMERGENCY ROOM IMMEDIATELY:

- New-onset numbness or weakness, particularly on one side of the face or body
- Sudden difficulty hearing, tasting, or swallowing
- Sudden problems moving the tongue
- Sudden dizziness or balance problems
- New-onset difficulty speaking or slurred speech
- New-onset problems walking or moving

brain (carotid endarterectomy or stenting) may be beneficial.

For long-term treatment, a stroke patient may be placed on blood thinners to lessen his chance of having another stroke. Depending on the injury that the stroke has caused, physical and occupational therapy can help improve an area of weakness. Speech and language therapy can help you regain the ability to speak. While most recovery happens within the first six months of having a stroke, people have been known to improve even after that window. Keeping up with a healthy diet and regular exercise during the healing period can help maximize your recovery from stroke.

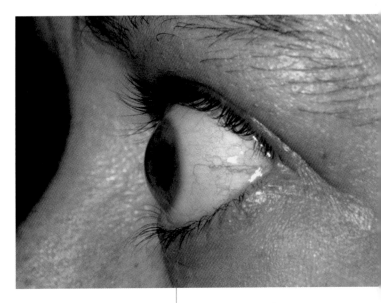

The bulging eye of a person with thyroid disease. The soft tissue in the eye socket has swollen, forcing the eye forward.

Thyroid disease

People with thyroid eye disease often have a typical appearance with one or both eyes that bulge forward. This happens because thyroid gland dysfunction causes inflammation and swelling in the tissues in the orbit, which then pushes the eyeballs forward. Usually the thyroid is overactive, as in Graves' Disease, but in some cases the thyroid can be underactive or even secrete normal amounts of thyroid hormone.

Signs of thyroid eye disease also include:

- Dry eye syndrome due to poor eyelid closure.
- Eye redness and irritation caused by dryness and congestion of the tissue.
- Double vision caused by inflammation and misalignment of the muscles that move the eyeballs.
- Optic nerve damage from compression of the inflamed tissues in the orbit.

If your eye doctor suspects that you have thyroid eye disease, she will refer you to your family doctor to check your thyroid hormone levels. If these levels are abnormal, you'll be treated for thyroid disease. Normalizing these hormone levels may help to stabilize the eye involvement, but there are also specific treatments for the eye problems themselves. If the eye disease is mild and dryness is the main problem, using artificial teardrops for lubrication or possibly lubricating gel or ointment in your eyes at bedtime may help. More severe disease that causes extremely dry eyes or optic nerve damage may be treated by oral steroid medicines, radiation, or surgery to decompress the orbit and

QUESTIONS TO ASK YOUR EYE DOCTOR

If you have thyroid eye disease:

- Is my eye disease mild enough so that my symptoms are just a nuisance?
- Or is my disease severe enough that my vision and the health of my eyes are at risk?

make more space for the inflamed, congested tissues. Once the eye disease has stabilized, any misalignment of the eyeballs that causes double vision can be corrected with eye muscle surgery or with prisms in your eyeglasses. Also, eyelids that have an abnormal position, which can contribute to the bulging appearance of the eyes, can then be repositioned with eyelid surgery if necessary.

Although there's nothing that you can do to prevent thyroid disease and its eye problems from occurring, there are steps you can take to help the course of the disease. If you suspect that you or someone else has signs of thyroid eye disease, consult an eye doctor or family doctor promptly. Diagnosing the disease early may mean that treatment is simpler and more likely to be successful. Don't smoke if you have thyroid eye disease, as smoking makes the disease worse. While severe vision loss from thyroid eye disease is fortunately rare, the way in which it can affect your appearance, and the double vision and dryness it can cause are more common. Luckily the treatments available for these problems can often help sufferers to maintain eye comfort as well as good vision.

Autoimmune diseases

Autoimmune diseases are those in which your body mistakenly sees certain aspects of itself as foreign. Therefore your body's immune system fights against itself, which causes the disease. There are a number of autoimmune diseases that all involve this type of dysfunction of the immune system. Examples of these diseases include: systemic lupus erythematosus, rheumatoid arthritis, sarcoidosis, ankylosing spondylitis, and Sjogren's syndrome.

Not everyone with an autoimmune disease develops eye problems because of it, but in many cases, autoimmune diseases cause dry eye syndrome. This happens because the disease makes the lacrimal, or tear gland, inflamed so that it can't produce tears normally. Also, just as other parts of the body can be inflamed, the eyes can also develop inflammation caused by autoimmune diseases. Uveitis, scleritis, and episcleritis are all terms that describe inflammation in various parts of the eyeball that can be caused by autoimmune diseases. If you suffer from one of these types of eye inflammation, you may notice eye pain, redness, light sensitivity, or decreased vision.

Treatment of eye inflammation from autoimmune disease has two goals. First,

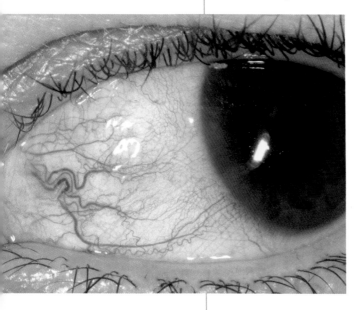

Inflammation of the sclera, the white part of the eye. This is often caused by an autoimmune disease.

the underlying disease needs to be controlled as well as possible; your eye doctor will refer you to a rheumatologist or internist for this. There have been many recent strides forward in the drugs available to treat autoimmune problems, so many people do quite well with proper medications. Second, your eye doctor will help you target the eye involvement. Steroid eyedrops and possibly oral or injectable steroid medicines may be used for the eye inflammation.

There is nothing you can do to reduce your risk of developing autoimmune diseases. It's not known what causes this type of disease, although in many cases they seem to run in families. If you notice eye symptoms of pain, redness, light sensitivity, or decreased vision, see your eye doctor promptly, since treating the cause of these problems early can lead to better long-term vision and better eye health.

> People who are chronically treated with steroid medicines for autoimmune diseases should have regular eye exams to screen for cataracts and glaucoma.

Migraine

Did you know that migraine headaches can affect your vision? Migraine is a brain disorder that can lead to headaches as well as to neurologic or mood disturbances. Up to 34 percent of women aged 15–20 have experienced at least one migraine, making this an extremely common problem that tends to affect women more than men. No one knows for sure what exactly causes migraine, although the disorder tends to run in families. Common theories state that the brain releases chemicals in response to a stressor and that those chemicals cause blood vessel constriction and pain. If you have suffered from a migraine, you may be prone to developing another in the future, although this is widely variable and depends on the person.

Migraine headaches tend to be throbbing, may be located on one side of the head, and are often associated with sensitivity to light and sound as well as nausea and sometimes even vomiting. Some people notice an aura prior to developing a migraine headache. An aura is an unusual smell, sound, or visual change that serves as a warning sign that a migraine is happening. One classic type of aura that affects vision is seeing flashing lights, blind spots, or bright zigzag lines in your side vision. This type of visual aura can sometimes occur without a headache afterward; if so, it is called an ocular migraine.

Migraines usually last for minutes to hours. In the vast majority of cases, the vision changes

COMMON MIGRAINE TRIGGERS INCLUDE

- Certain food or drink, such as chocolate or alcohol
- Stress
- Changes in sleep habits
- Hormonal fluctuations
- Medications
- Smoke exposure
- Changes in the weather

and neurologic changes go away completely after each episode and leave no lasting effects. Very rarely, someone with migraines may suffer a permanent neurologic defect from the migraine.

There are many medications available to prevent and treat migraines. If you suffer from severe or frequent migraines, see your family doctor or neurologist to find out which of these treatments can help you. Migraines can also be prevented to some extent by getting enough sleep as well as regular exercise, which help reduce stress and tension. Another thing you can do is find out if your migraine is triggered by anything in particular. Keeping track of these triggers in a diary, along with the timing of when your migraines occur, may help you pinpoint a cause, and then you can take care to avoid that particular trigger as much as you can.

Sexually transmitted diseases

Sexually transmitted diseases (STDs) can also affect your eyes. Examples are human immunodeficiency virus (HIV), gonorrhea, chlamydia, herpes, human papilloma virus, and syphilis. While these diseases cause eye problems in different ways, all can cause inflammation in or around the eyes.

HIV can cause eye problems when the disease is severe and the CD4 count is less than 300 cells/μl. Therefore, in the early stages of HIV infection, you can have a normal eye exam. HIV, when it does affect the eyes, most commonly causes inflammation in the retina in intermediate and advanced stages of the disease. This may affect your vision but can also help make the diagnosis of HIV if the eye doctor sees signs of inflammation and can't find any other cause. In the later stages of HIV infection, other infections can take advantage of the weakened immune system and cause eye problems. These types of infections in the front part of the eye include Kaposi sarcoma, which can cause growths on your eyelids and conjunctiva, and herpes simplex and herpes zoster viruses, which can affect your cornea and the front part of your eyeball, as well as your retina. Other infections that can damage your retina and result in vision loss in people with advanced HIV include cytomegalovirus, toxoplasma, candida, cryptococcus, and pneumocystis.

Gonorrhea and chlamydia are two STDs that can also affect the health of your eyes. If the bacteria that cause these diseases touch the eye, they can cause conjunctivitis, or inflammation of the conjunctiva. Gonorrhea, in particular, tends to progress quickly and be very aggressive if it causes an eye infection, and it can even lead to severe vision loss in some situations. For this reason, all newborns are generally treated with antibiotic eye ointment at the time of birth to prevent infections from any gonorrhea or chlamydia bacteria that might be present in the mother as the newborn passes through the birth canal.

Genital herpes belongs to the herpes family of viruses, which has many members. Herpes simplex virus type 2, in particular, tends to cause genital blisters and lesions. While genital herpes viruses do not affect your eyes as commonly as other types of the herpes virus, these type 2 viruses can cause inflammation (uveitis) in the front or back parts of your eyeball. These infections tend to be more severe overall than eye infections caused by other types of herpes viruses.

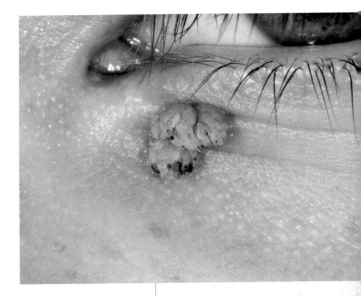

Human papilloma virus is a family of viruses that include those responsible for genital warts and cervical cancer and can also affect your eyes by causing warts on your eyelids or on the surface of your eyeball. These warts generally do not cause major vision problems, but they can be unsightly and may cause eye irritation. Depending on the location of the warts, they can be removed with surgery and medicines, but they may recur in the future.

Warts are harmless, contagious growths on the outermost layer of the skin (epidermis). They are caused by the human papilloma virus (HPV).

Syphilis is a bacterium that has caused disease for centuries, and although its infections are not as common as they once were before the era of antibiotics, they still occur. Syphilis can either be acquired by sexual contact or passed from a pregnant woman to her unborn child. It starts as a genital infection; if untreated, it can spread all over the body and cause eye disease in its later stages. Nearly every part of your eye is susceptible to developing inflammation from syphilis. Fortunately, syphilis is treatable with antibiotics, but the eye inflammation it can cause may result in long-term damage to your vision even after treatment.

While the sexually transmitted diseases that can cause eye problems are all treatable, prevention is the best way to avoid these troubling disorders.

All of the STDs that can cause eye problems have two things in commmon: they are preventable, and if you do develop one or more of them, they are treatable. However, since many of the eye problems caused by STDs can damage the vision permanently even if they are treated, avoiding these diseases in the first place is the best option. High-risk sexual behavior exposes you to STDs and all their associated problems. In the case of HIV, sharing needles is another method of transmission. Using condoms decreases, but does not eliminate, the chance of contracting an STD, and so it is best to take all precautions.

5

Eye Comfort

Despite its relatively small size, the front surface of the eye has one of the highest concentrations of nerve fibers in the entire body. Even a small corneal abrasion from getting poked in the eye can be tremendously uncomfortable and can result in tearing, redness, and pain. There are many reasons why patients experience ocular discomfort, but there are ways of alleviating such discomfort.

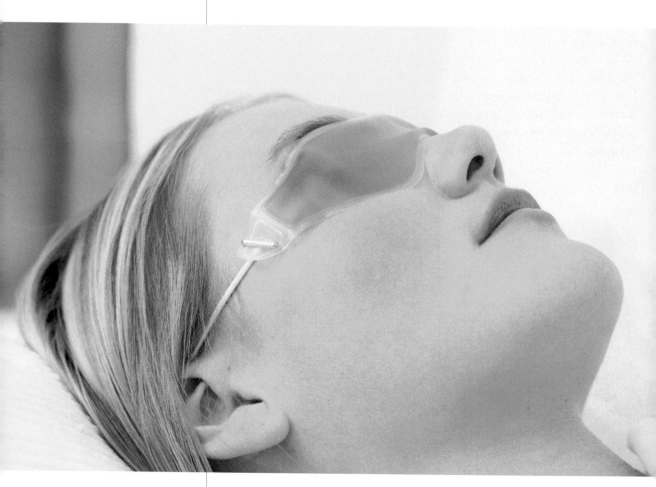

Tearing

Excessive tearing can be due to one of two problems—either the eye is producing more tears than are necessary, or the tear duct that drains the tears is not functioning properly. The overproduction of tears can be due to several causes, including allergic reaction, infection on the eye surface or within the eye, inflammation on the eye surface or in the eye, or irritation caused by excessive dryness or an injury to the eye. The eyes can also be stimulated to make extra tears when a person is crying.

Allergic conjunctivitis

To help understand what is causing an eye to water too much, it is helpful to try to determine the specific circumstances that trigger the eyes to start tearing and identify other symptoms associated with the tearing. For example allergic conjunctivitis is an allergic reaction to certain substances in the environment. When exposed to substances such as pollen, mold, dust, or animal dander, your eyes can become irritated and inflamed. (See chapter 3 for further information).

Viral conjunctivitis

Another frequent cause of tearing is an infection on the surface of the eye, such as viral conjunctivitis. Commonly called pinkeye, viral conjunctivitis is a highly contagious condition that can spread easily from one person to another. It often starts in one eye and within seven to ten days spreads to the other eye; it can take up to two weeks for the infection to resolve in both eyes. A person who develops pinkeye often knows other people at home or work who are having symptoms similar to theirs. These symptoms include excessive tearing with a watery discharge, redness of the eye, and a foreign-body sensation—that is, feeling as though there is sand or some other substance in your eyes that

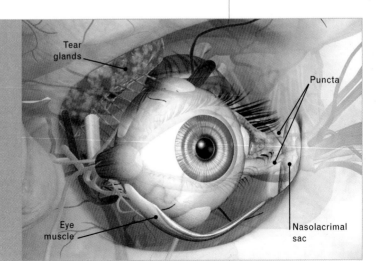

THE LACRIMAL DRAINAGE SYSTEM

The tears that bathe the front surface of the eye are produced in the lacrimal gland, which is situated behind the upper eyelid. When a person blinks, the eyelids help push the tears across the eye surface. They collect in the lower inner corner of the eye. They travel through the puncta, into the lacrimal sac, and down the nasolacrimal duct into the nose and down the throat.

Tear glands

Puncta

Eye muscle

Nasolacrimal sac

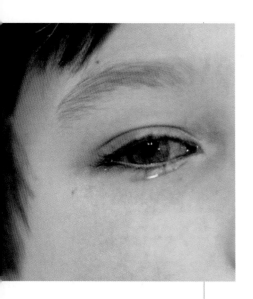

does not belong there. Although this condition can make the eyes feel uncomfortable, vision is usually not affected. The same virus that causes pinkeye can affect the upper respiratory tract, causing fever and a sore throat.

Dry eyes

Interestingly tearing is often caused by excessive dryness of the eyes. When the eyes get dried out, a reflex that causes the lacrimal gland (the gland that produces tears) to make more tears is triggered. Sometimes this occurs when a person is reading for long periods of time and becomes so focused on his reading material that he forgets to blink regularly. Understanding why the eyes have become so dry and treating the source of the dryness with artificial tears or other lubricants can be useful.

A young boy with viral conjunctivitis. Note the redness of the eye and the watery discharge.

Corneal abrasion

A variety of different injuries to the eye can cause excessive tearing. A very common eye injury is a corneal abrasion that occurs when the superficial cells on the front surface of the eye become damaged. This can happen from being poked in the eye, having a foreign body come in contact with the front surface of the eye, or vigorously rubbing the eye. Because the cornea is one of the most sensitive organs in the entire body, the surface cells can feel really uncomfortable when damaged. Symptoms associated with corneal abrasions include profuse tearing; a foreign-body sensation in the eye; redness of the eye; sensitivity to light; and, if the damaged cells are at or close to the center of the cornea, blurry vision. Small abrasions usually heal quickly (in 1 or 2 days), whereas larger abrasions can take up to a week or longer to heal completely. If your eye is injured, you should contact your eye doctor, as he or she can examine the eye to check for possible infection and make sure that only the superficial cells of the cornea were affected by the injury. Antibiotics can be prescribed to prevent infection until the abrasion has healed completely.

OPTICAL ILLUSION

It was once thought that placing a patch over the eye would be helpful with corneal abrasions because it would help the eye heal and prevent infection. But studies have shown that simple corneal abrasions heal more quickly without the use of a patch. Also, wearing a patch over the eye can actually hide the presence of an infection that could delay treatment. Thus patching the eye is not recommended for most corneal abrasions.

Foreign bodies

A foreign body, such as a torn contact lens, a chemical substance sprayed accidently in the eye, or even one's own eyelash, can irritate the eye and cause tearing with every blink. Whenever a foreign substance gets in the eye, the eye must be washed out immediately with plenty of water to try to dislodge the substance or remove as much of the irritant as possible before it can seep further into the eye. Next, you should immediately contact your eye doctor so that he or she can examine the eye for possible damage. Foreign bodies that get embedded in the cornea may not become dislodged with irrigation alone and may need to be removed by an eye care professional.

Other causes of tearing

Tearing can be associated with a few serious, sight-threatening conditions. When tearing is accompanied by blurry vision that does not improve by simply wiping away the excess tears, you should have your eyes examined by an eye doctor to be sure that you do not have conditions such as acute angle-closure glaucoma or uveitis. Angle-closure glaucoma occurs when the drain that normally removes excess fluid from the eye becomes blocked, and the eye pressure suddenly gets very high. Patients experience tearing, redness, tremendous pain around the eye, blurry vision, nausea, and vomiting. If the eye pressure is not lowered immediately, the nerve can be permanently damaged, causing irreversible vision loss. In contrast to conjunctivitis, in which the inflammation occurs on the surface of the eye, uveitis is inflammation that occurs inside the eye. Individuals with uveitis can experience blurry vision, redness, sensitivity to light, tearing, and eye pain. If untreated, this condition can damage the structures in the eye. Excessive tearing in an infant also requires a thorough eye examination to make sure he or she does not have a vision-threatening condition like congenital glaucoma.

> There is no connection between the tears that bathe the surface of the eye and the fluid that is located within the eye.

Blocked tear ducts in newborns

Blockage of the tear ducts is a common cause of tearing in newborns. Normally the tears bathe the front surface of the eye and then travel through the tear ducts, into the nose and down the throat. To keep the tears flowing

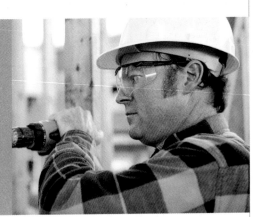

SAFETY GOGGLES

A simple way to prevent foreign bodies from getting into the eye is to wear safety goggles when working with drills, saws, or other construction equipment that creates the release of debris into the air. For those who wear glasses, prescription goggles are also available.

True or False?
Blockage of the tear duct in infants is uncommon, affecting only 1 in 6,000 babies.

False

Blockage of the tear duct is actually quite common in babies, affecting 6 of every 100 (6 percent).

properly in the correct direction (so they do not flow backward from the nose back into the eye), there are small valves that are present in the tear ducts. Normally, these valves open up around the time of birth. However, for some babies, the valves remain closed for awhile after birth. If the valves are not yet open, the tears cannot drain properly. They accumulate on the surface of the eye and can run down the cheek. In the majority of babies who have blocked tear ducts at birth, the valves will open up spontaneously within the first year of life, allowing the tears to drain properly. For babies with blocked tear ducts, parents are encouraged to massage the skin overlying the tear ducts to help speed up the opening of the valves. If this does not solve the problem and tearing persists, an ophthalmologist can perform a probing procedure that will open up the tear ducts and correct the tearing.

Blocked tear ducts in adults

Blockage of the tear ducts is an uncommon cause of tearing in adults. Over time, scar tissue can develop within the tear duct, limiting the ability of the tears to flow through properly. Conditions that can lead to scar tissue buildup in the tear ducts include infections that develop within the tear duct, injury to the tear duct, medications that can irritate the tear duct, and cancer of the tear duct. Often when adults experience blockage of the tear ducts, the condition, unlike with infants, does not usually resolve itself. Correcting the obstruction often requires an ophthalmologist inserting silicone tubes through the tear duct into the nose to create a new pathway for the tears to exit the surface of the eye. If there is too much scar tissue to fit silicone tubes through the tear ducts, sometimes the ophthalmologist must perform surgery to create a new pathway for the tears to flow from the eye into the nose. This surgery is called dacrocystorhinostomy.

Dry eyes

For several reasons it is important to maintain an adequate amount of tears to coat the surface of the eye. The tears serve a protective function. They wash away debris that gathers on the surface of the eye, including bacteria and other microorganisms, allergens, and irritating chemicals that can damage the cornea. Moreover, tears contain antibodies to help prevent infection. Tears carry nutrients to the cells on the surface of the cornea and remove corneal cells when they become damaged or die. If debris collects on the corneal surface, it can affect how light enters the eye and result in blurry vision. Tears keep debris away from the cornea; this allows light to enter the eye undisturbed, which is necessary for clear vision.

It is estimated that more than 20 million Americans have dry eyes.

The front surface of the eye can be compared to the windshield of a car.

In this analogy, the eyelids function as the windshield wipers, and the tears are like the windshield wiper fluid that washes away debris on the glass surface. Just as it would be difficult without windshield wipers or windshield wiper fluid for a driver to see through the windshield when dirt or debris collect on its surface, it is difficult to see if there are problems with the eyelids or tear production.

Tears are made up of oil, water, and mucins (heavily glycosylated proteins). The largest component of the tear film is water, which is produced continuously by the lacrimal glands. Emotional, painful, or noxious stimuli can trigger the lacrimal gland to secrete even more of this component. The conjunctiva produces mucins that help the tears flow across the surface of the eye. The final component is a thin layer of oil that prevents the tears from drying up as they move across the surface of the eye. The oily layer is produced by the meibomian glands, which are located on the eyelids. Deficiencies in any of these components can cause abnormal tears that fail to bathe the surface of the eye and keep it comfortable and seeing clearly.

> Patients who have blepharitis are prone to developing painful bumps on the surface of the eyelids known as sties.

Causes of dry eyes

When evaluating a patient for dry eyes, the eye doctor can assess whether there are abnormalities in any of these components of the tears. Various conditions can damage the lacrimal gland and affect its ability to secrete the watery component of the tears. Medical conditions such as sarcoidosis, lupus, and the Sjögren syndrome can inflame the lacrimal gland, causing it to function improperly. In addition, several systemic medications (medications used to treat medical conditions unrelated to the eye) can affect the amount of secretions produced by the lacrimal gland. Dry eye is a potential side effect of all the medications listed in the table on the next page.

Since the mucinous component of the tear film is produced by the conjunctiva, any eye condition or other medical condition that damages the conjunctiva can affect the amount of mucin in the tears and result in dry eyes. Examples of conditions that can cause damage to the conjunctiva include chemical injuries (that is, when acids or alkali substances get in the eye), vitamin A deficiency, autoimmune and other medical conditions that damage mucosal surfaces throughout the body.

Dry eyes commonly result from abnormalities of the lipid layer of the tear film. When the oil glands get plugged up, a condition known as meibomianitis or blepharitis, they

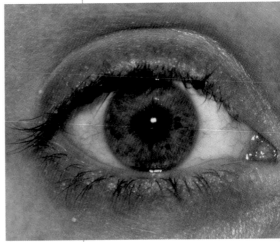

Photograph of a patient with blepharitis.
Notice the redness and inflammation of the eyelids and the buildup of crust on the eyelashes.

MEDICATIONS WITH DRY EYE AS A SIDE EFFECT

Acebutolol
Acetophenazine
Albuterol
Aluminum nicotinate
Amitriptyline
Antazoline
Atenolol
Atropine
Azatadine

Belladonna
Bendroflumethiazide
Benzalkonium
Benzthiazide
Brimonidine tartrate
Brompheniramine
Busulfan
Butaperazine

Carbinoxamine
Carphenazine
Chlorisondamine
Chlorothiazide
Chlorpheniramine
Chlorpromazine
Chlorthalidone
Clemastine
Clonidine
Cyclothiazide
Cyproheptadine

Desipramine
Dexbrompheniramine
Dexchlorpheniramine
Diethazine
Dimethindene
Diphenhydramine
Diphenylpyraline
Disopyramide
Doxylamine
Dronabinol

Emedastine difumarate
Ether
Ethopropazine
Etretinate

Fluphenazine

Hashish
Hexamethonium
Homatropine
Hydrochlorothiazide
Hydroflumethiazide

Imipramine
Indapamide
Isotretinoin

Labetolol
Lithium carbonate

Marijuana
Mesoridazine
Methdilazine
Methotrexate
Methotrimeprazine
Methoxsalen
Methscopolamine
Methyclothiadize
Methylthiouracil
Metolazone
Metoprolol
Morphine

Nadolol
Niacin
Niacinamide
Nicotinyl alcohol
Nitrous oxide
Nortriptyline

Opium
Oxprenolol

Pentazocine
Perazine
Periciazine
Perphenazine
Pheniramine
Pimozide
Pindolol
Piperacetazine
Polythiazide
Practolol
Prochlorperazine
Promazine
Promethazine
Propiomazine
Propranolol
Protriptyline
Pyrilamine

Quinethazone

Scopolamine

Tetrahydrocannabinol
THC
Thiethylperazine
Thiopropazate
Thioproperazine
Thioridazine
Timolol
Tolterodine tartrate
Trichlormethiazide
Trichloroethylene
Trifluoperazine
Triflupromazine
Trimeprazine
Trioxsalen
Tripelennamine
Triprolidine

Reprinted from: Fraunfelder, FT and Fraunfelder FW. Drug-Induced Ocular Side Effects, 5th edition, Butterworth Heinemann, Boston, MA, 2001, p 654-655.

cannot adequately secrete the oily layer of the tears that prevents the tears from evaporating. In addition to dry eyes, people with blepharitis commonly experience redness; a gritty sensation; and crust that builds up on the surface of the eye, which is especially noticeable on awakening in the morning.

Finally, dry eyes can be caused by problems with the functioning of the eyelids. Just as seeing through a car windshield when it is raining would be difficult if the windshield wipers were broken, portions of the surface of the eye will become dry if the eyelids cannot properly push the tears across the surface of the eye. Scarring of the eyelids from prior inflammation, infection, or injuries can alter the shape of the eyelids or their ability to open and close properly. Damage to the nerves that control the eyelids, due to conditions such as Bell's palsy can also prevent the eyelids from functioning properly. Conditions like Graves' disease, which results from hyperthyroidism, can cause the eyeball to protrude forward from the eye socket, making it difficult for the eyelids to push the tears across the eye surface. When a person is reading for a prolonged period of time and becomes engrossed in the material, he may forget to blink often enough. This can result in blurry vision due to dryness.

> Periodic use of artificial tears can soothe the eye and improve vision in patients who have excessively dry eyes.

Determining why your eyes are dry

Since there are a multitude of different conditions that can cause dry eyes, if you are bothered by dry eyes, you should speak with an eye doctor, who can thoroughly assess whether any systemic medical or ocular conditions may be contributing to your dry eyes. The doctor can also review any medications you may be taking to determine if any of them

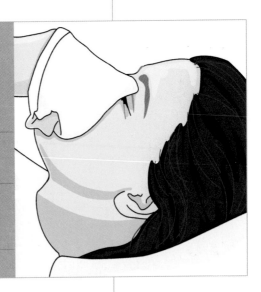

BLEPHARITIS

If you have blepharitis, performing these simple steps can keep your eyes feeling more comfortable. You may need to perform them regularly in order to notice a benefit (generally twice daily is recommended).

- Wring a clean washcloth out under warm tap water.

- Close your eyes and put the washcloth on your eyelids for 3–5 minutes. This helps to loosen any clogged oil glands and normalize the oil layer of your tear film.

- Afterward, put a tiny drop of tear-free baby shampoo on the washcloth and gently massage your eyelids while your eyes are closed. This will help remove any crusting and bacteria at the base of your eyelids.

- Rinse thoroughly to wash away surface debris.

might be causing or exacerbating the dryness. In addition they can evaluate all of the ocular structures, including the eyelids, the conjunctiva, and the cornea, to look for clues to determine why your eyes are dry and to make sure that the cornea is not developing damage because of persistent dryness. Finally, they can perform tests in the office to determine whether your lacrimal gland is producing enough tears and obtain a sample of the tears to check for abnormalities in specific components of the tear film.

What can I do to help my dry eyes?

The most effective way to treat dry eyes is to target the specific conditions causing the dryness. For example, if your dryness is primarily due to the use of a medication, the dryness may improve if you can reduce or discontinue use of the drug or switch to an alternative medication (your eye doctor can advise you on this). If the main cause of your dryness is related to blepharitis, using warm compresses to open up the plugged oil glands and cleaning the eyelid surface with diluted baby shampoo to wash away bacteria and

TREATMENTS FOR DRY EYES

TYPE OF EYEDROP	WHEN TO USE	COMMENTS
Artificial tears	As often as you like to help dry eye symptoms. If you use more than 4 times per day, consider using preservative-free artificial tears.	Many brands are available over the counter. If you use medicated eyedrops for another eye disease, wait at least five minutes after using the medicated drop before instilling an artificial teardrop.
Preservative-free artificial tears	As often as you like for dry eye symptoms. Especially good for people with sensitivities to preservatives or for those who use teardrops more than 4 times per day.	More expensive than artificial tears containing preservatives.
Lubricating gels	May be best used at bedtime, depending on your preference.	Gels are thicker than artificial tears and so may blur your vision more.
Lubricating ointments	Best used at bedtime.	Ointments are thicker than artificial tears and lubricating gels, so they will blur your vision.

secretions plugging up the oil glands can significantly improve the symptoms. In addition to treating the conditions or factors causing the dryness, most patients with dry eyes experience relief of their symptoms with the use of artificial tears and other eye lubricants. Many brands of artificial tears are sold over the counter.

In addition to using artificial tears, some patients with dry eyes may benefit from using lubricating ointments at bedtime to keep the surface of the eye from drying out. If use of lubricating eyedrops or ointments alone is ineffective, you should speak with your eye doctor to ask whether you may benefit from additional treatments, such as cyclosporine eyedrops (Restasis) or temporary blockage of the tear duct with a punctal plug.

Itchy eyes

Many of the same conditions that can result in excessive tearing of the eyes are also associated with itchy eyes. These conditions include allergic conjunctivitis, viral conjunctivitis (pinkeye), blepharitis, and dry eyes (descriptions of each of these conditions can be found in chapter 3). To determine which of these conditions is causing your itchy eyes, it is helpful to know how long you have been bothered by the itchy eyes, what other symptoms are accompanying the itchy eyes, and whether the itchy eyes are worse in certain environments. Conditions such as blepharitis and dry eyes are often long-standing conditions that, if left untreated, can continually irritate the eye and cause it to itch throughout the year, perhaps even longer. Allergic conjunctivitis often flares up during certain seasons of the year or after exposure to triggers like dust, pollen, or grass. Itchiness caused by pinkeye occurs suddenly and often resolves completely within three weeks, as the virus clears your system.

For people with mildly itchy eyes, storing artificial teardrops in the refrigerator can make them especially soothing when you use them.

What can I do to stop my eyes from itching?

The appropriate treatment for itchy eyes depends on the cause. In addition to treatments aimed at the cause of the itchiness (see the section above on tearing for descriptions of treatments for each of these conditions), various medications can be used to target and reduce the itchiness. Various types of prescription eyedrops (for example, levocabastine, emedastine, antazoline, naphazoline, lodoxamide, olopatadine, cromolyn) can reduce itchiness caused by allergies. Antihistamines taken by mouth can also be useful in patients with allergic conjunctivitis. In severe cases, corticosteroid eyedrops may be necessary to relieve the symptoms of allergic conjunctivitis.

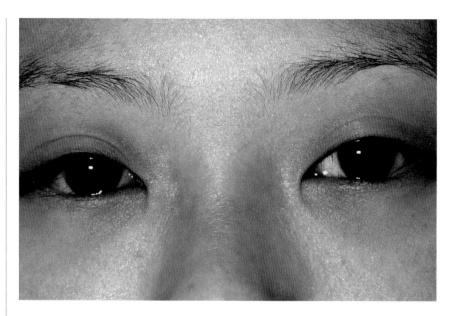

Allergic conjunctivitis is characterized by swelling and puffiness of the eyelids, redness and irritation of the conjunctiva, and watering of the eyes. A prominent symptom of allergic conjunctivitis is itching.

Eye pain

Several types of ocular conditions can cause eye pain. Eye pain can result from serious, potentially sight-threatening ocular conditions or from relatively minor conditions. The following questions will help your eye doctor identify the source of the pain:

- How would you describe the pain? Is it a sharp pain, a dull ache, a throbbing sensation?
- How long does the pain last?
- Is the pain continuous or intermittent?
- Do any specific activities cause the pain to get worse or make the pain go away?
- What other symptoms accompany the pain?
- Have you ever had eye surgery?
- Do you wear contact lenses?

Serious ocular conditions known to cause eye pain include acute angle-closure glaucoma, corneal ulcer (an infection to the surface of the eye), endophthalmitis (an infection within the eye), uveitis, scleritis, and optic neuritis (inflammation of different structures within the eye). Less serious conditions known to cause eye pain include corneal abrasions, trichiasis (when eyelashes turn inward, causing them to rub up against the front surface of eye), conjunctivitis, blepharitis, and dry eyes.

Patients who experience an abrupt loss of vision along with their eye pain should urgently visit their eye doctor for an evaluation to make sure they do not have a serious condition that can permanently damage the eye. Patients at increased risk for infections on the surface of or within their eyes, including patients who have had a recent injury to their eyes, recent surgery on their eyes, those who wear contact lenses, and those with medical conditions that compromise the function of their immune system, should also see an eye doctor if they experience pain in their eyes. A thorough eye exam by your eye doctor will usually identify the source of the pain. Since different conditions that cause eye pain are treated differently, once the source of the pain is identified, the eye doctor can prescribe the appropriate medications to help alleviate the symptoms.

Headaches

More than 45 million Americans are believed to suffer from chronic headaches. According to the World Health Organization, 1 in every 20 persons living in developed countries experiences chronic, daily headaches.

Why am I getting headaches?

People can get headaches for various reasons. To help your physician determine why you are experiencing headaches, you should try to provide him or her with as much information about the nature of the headache as you can. The following questions can be helpful in determining the cause:

- When you get a headache, what part of your head hurts?
- Each time you get a headache, is it always the same part of the head that hurts, or does it vary from one episode to the next?
- How long do your headaches usually last?
- How often do you experience headaches?
- What makes your headaches feel worse?
- What makes your headaches feel better (for example, sleeping, taking non-prescription pain relievers)?
- Are there certain activities or circumstances that seem to trigger your headaches?
- Do you experience other symptoms, such as weakness, blurry vision, or nausea, along with the headache?

Overuse of certain medications to treat migraine headaches may actually cause a worsening of the migraine symptoms when the medication is discontinued, a phenomenon known as a rebound effect.

Tension headaches

A tension headache is the most common type of headache, accounting for 90 percent of all headaches; it is characterized as a dull persistent ache. Some patients describe the sensation as having a band tied tightly around their head. These headaches are commonly associated with physical or emotional stressors and can last from less than one hour up to several days.

TEST YOUR
Eye Q:

True or False?

Common causes of eye pain include cataracts, open-angle glaucoma, and macular degeneration.

False

In general, pain is not a major feature of any of these common eye conditions.

Migraine headaches

Migraines are another common form of headache, affecting roughly 12 percent of the population. Migraines tend to run in families, and they are more common among females than males.

Unlike tension headaches, a migraine is characterized by intense throbbing pain, often affecting one side of the head; it lasts 4–72 hours. The headache is accompanied by sensitivity to light and sound and is frequently associated with nausea and vomiting. Approximately 20 percent of patients who get migraine experience a visual aura lasting 20–40 minutes before the headache starts. The typical aura consists of flashing lights or zigzagging lines that start in one portion of the visual field, slowly expand to affect the center of the vision, and then "march" out to the periphery of the visual field before breaking up. There are a number of foods and environmental factors that can trigger migraines (see text box on page 114).

Treatments for migraine headaches include medications aimed at stopping an ongoing attack (abortive agents) and those that can prevent new attacks from occurring (preventive agents). Abortive agents include non-prescription pain relievers and two classes of prescription products—triptans and ergotamine derivatives. Over-the-counter pain relievers, such as aspirin, ibuprofen, and acetaminophen, can be effective at alleviating various types of mild headaches. When these non-prescription agents are ineffective, triptans and ergotamine derivatives can successfully relieve the pain during an acute migraine attack.

Patients who develop severe migraine headaches or experience frequent migraine headaches (more than one per week) may benefit from taking preventive agents. While these agents will not provide any pain relief during an acute attack, if taken regularly they can reduce the frequency and severity of future attacks. Preventive agents include drug classes called beta-blockers, calcium-channel blockers, antidepressants, and anticonvulsants.

Cluster headaches

Cluster headaches are an uncommon type of headache that usually affect males in their thirties and forties. These headaches tend to occur in cyclical patterns, with periods when the headaches occur frequently and other periods when there are none at all. People who get these headaches describe the pain as excruciating, as if someone has stuck a hot poker in the affected eye. The pain lasts 30 minutes to 3 hours and can be so uncomfortable that the patient may pace back and forth until the pain subsides. Associated symptoms are tearing and a runny nose on the same side of the face as the headache. Triggers associated with cluster headaches include drinking alcoholic beverages, smoking cigarettes, and having sleep disturbances. Treatments include breathing 100 percent oxygen and taking medications similar to those used for migraine headaches (for example, sumatriptan and dihydroergotamine).

Experts have described the pain associated with cluster headaches as the most severe pain known to medical science. Some women describe the pain as more severe than childbirth.

Sinus headaches

The sinuses are air-filled cavities located in the forehead, around the eyes, and over the cheeks. Normally, mucus accumulates in the sinuses and drains into the nose. Sinus headaches are caused by obstruction of the affected sinus by inflammation, infection (sinusitis), or other causes. When the sinus cannot properly drain, fluid builds up and causes a dull, constant, aching pain over the affected sinus. This discomfort can be accompanied by fever, nasal discharge, or facial swelling. If your doctor suspects you have sinusitis, she may obtain a CT (Computed Tomography) scan to more thoroughly investigate whether the sinuses are obstructed before beginning treatment with antibiotics and decongestants.

Headaches due to eyestrain

Eyestrain is a common cause of headaches or achy eyes. Patients experience discomfort if they are wearing an incorrect eye glass prescription or if their eyes are not working properly together. For example, when a person with myopia (nearsightedness) is undercorrected (that is, her glasses or contact lens prescription is not strong enough), she may try to see more clearly by narrowing her eyes. Maintaining this position for prolonged periods of time can result in headaches or eyestrain. Another example is when a person with hyperopia (farsightedness) loses

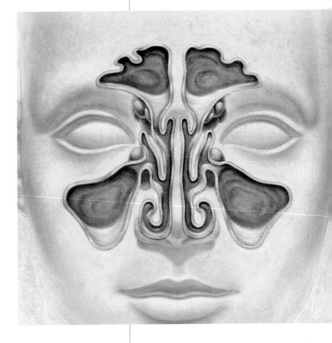

The sinuses (colored in red) are situated around the eyes and nose. Obstruction of the sinuses can lead to sinus headaches.

RISK FACTORS FOR DEVELOPING SINUS HEADACHES

- History of hay fever or seasonal allergies
- High altitudes
- Frequent swimming
- Blockage of the nasal passage by growths of tissue known as nasal polyps

True or False?

People can have symptoms of migraines without the headache.

True

As one gets older, the frequency of migraine headaches often decreases, but a person can still experience the visual symptoms related to migraines without developing a headache; this is known as an acephalgic migraine.

his accommodation (that is, the ability to focus up close), which often occurs around the age of forty. Without the aid of reading spectacles, the extra effort exerted over a prolonged period by the eye muscles to keep the words on the page looking clear can cause eyestrain. In both these scenarios, receiving the correct eye glass prescription for one's vision should alleviate the symptoms. A third example occurs when the muscles that control the movements of the two eyes are unbalanced. Prolonged effort exerted by the eye muscles to keep the eyes working together without experiencing double vision can result in eyestrain. In this case, the patient often experiences intermittent double vision at the end of the day, when the eye muscles become tired.

Temporal arteritis

Also known as giant cell arteritis or cranial arteritis, temporal arteritis is an uncommon but serious medical condition that, if left untreated, can result in irreversible blindness. This condition affects patients over the age of 50 years, and is characterized by inflammation affecting the

MIGRAINE HEADACHE TRIGGERS	
FOODS	• Alcohol • Caffeine (and caffeine withdrawal) • Citrus fruits, nuts, onions, peanut butter • Chocolate • Dairy products; aged cheeses • Foods containing monosodium glutamate; pickled or marinated foods • Meats containing nitrates (hot dogs, bacon)
OTHER	• Changes in the weather or season • Certain classes of drugs, including oral contraceptives, estrogen replacement therapy, nitrates, decongestants • Cigarette smoke • Flashing lights • Hunger • Intense physical exertion • Menstruation; menopause • Perfumes • Sun glare • Stress • Sleep disturbances (too little or too much sleep)

blood supply to the head and eyes. Patients with this condition complain of headaches that occur over the temples accompanied by pain when combing one's hair, or when trying to chew food. In addition, patients with temporal arteritis often have fever, night sweats, shoulder or hip pain, and weight loss. When the blood supply to the eye is affected, patients complain of transient vision loss.

Therefore, if you are experiencing the symptoms described above and suspect you might have this condition, you should contact your doctor or go to the hospital emergency room immediately. Temporal arteritis is usually treated with a high dose of corticosteroids.

If it is necessary for you to be treated for a prolonged period of time with corticosteroids, your doctor will need to monitor the level of intraocular pressure in your eyes, since the use of these medications can increase your risk of glaucoma.

Other causes of headaches

Although the majority of patients with headaches have one of the types of headache syndromes described above, some headaches are associated with serious medical conditions. The American Headache Society has compiled a list of symptoms (see below) that can suggest the possibility of a serious underlying medical condition requiring urgent evaluation and treatment. If you have any of these symptoms or conditions associated with your headache, you should contact your family doctor immediately. A list of support groups for people who suffer from migraine headaches can be found at the following website: www.migraines.org/help.

SYMPTOMS REQUIRING IMMEDIATE MEDICAL ATTENTION

- **First or worst headache of your life**
- **Abrupt onset of headache without any warning signs or buildup**
- **Fundamental change in the pattern of recurrent headaches**
- **Headache beginning at an atypical age:**
  5 years old or younger
  50 years old or older
- **The presence of cancer or HIV infection**
- **Pregnancy**
- **Abnormal result on physical examination**
- **Headache onset with seizure or syncope**
- **Headache onset with exertion, sexual activity, or squeezing (known as valsalva)**

Adapted from the American Headache Society

6

Natural Treatments for Eye Health

As people in countries such as the United States and Canada are living increasingly longer, it becomes even more important to find ways of keeping people's eyes from losing sight as they age. Various vitamins, minerals, and herbal supplements are used to keep the eyes working properly and protect against damage related to aging.

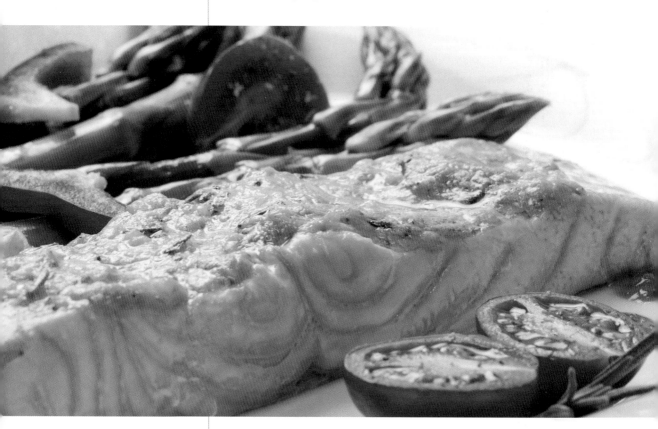

Key vitamins for eye health

Interest in using vitamins to maintain the health of the eye was sparked by a large study from the early 1990s called the Age-Related Eye Disease Study (AREDS). It involved over 4,500 patients at 11 healthcare centers across the United States. Some of the patients were given a supplement containing vitamins C and E, along with beta carotene, zinc, and copper, while others were given a placebo pill that lacked any vitamins or minerals. The patients were followed for approximately five years.

The researchers found that among the patients who had macular degeneration, those in the group getting vitamin and mineral supplements had a 25 percent lower chance of experiencing a worsening of their eye disease, compared with those receiving placebos. Scientists estimated that over a five-year period, 300,000 people with macular degeneration could be spared vision loss by taking supplements containing vitamins and consuming a diet rich in antioxidants.

Vitamin A

Vitamin A plays an important role in the health of the eye. In the front of the eye, vitamin A aids in the production of tears and helps lubricate the cornea and conjunctiva. Without high enough levels of this vitamin, the cornea—which is normally clear so that light can pass through it undisturbed to the back of the eye, allowing for sight—gets cloudy and the surface cells can break down. This can lead to infection and scarring that prevents light from entering the eye, eventually causing blindness. Vitamin A supports the rods in the retina at the back of the eye that are the photoreceptors responsible for night vision. In fact vitamin A consumed from animal sources is called retinol, a name that conveys the vitamin's importance to the retina.

Of all foods, liver contains the most vitamin A. High levels of vitamin A are also found in green leafy vegetables, fruit, eggs, butter, milk, and cheese. It's important to note that some sources of vitamin A are high in saturated fat and cholesterol, which can harm the body; so consuming excessive amounts of these foods is generally not advised.

TEST YOUR
Eye Q:

True or False?
There are a variety of causes for nyctalopia, or night blindness, one of which is a vitamin A deficiency.

True

FORMULATION OF VITAMINS AND SUPPLEMENTS USED IN AREDS

- 500 milligrams (mgs) of vitamin **C**
- 400 International Units (**IU**) of vitamin **E**
- 15 mgs of beta-carotene (often labeled as equivalent to 25,000 **IU** of vitamin **A**)
- 80 mgs of zinc as zinc oxide
- 2 mgs of copper as cupric oxide

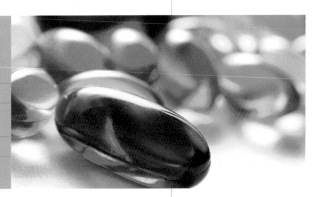

TEST YOUR
Eye Q:

True or False?
Cigarette smokers need one-and-a-half times the amount of vitamin C as nonsmokers.

True
Research suggests that people who are exposed to second-hand smoke may also need more vitamin C.

Vitamin A deficiency is a major cause of blindness in developing countries. The World Health Organization estimates that over 250,000 malnourished children go blind each year from this condition. Because vitamin A is important not only for eyesight but also for the immune system, unfortunately many children with this deficiency die if the condition goes untreated. Vitamin A deficiency can be easily treated with the right vitamin supplements.

Hypervitaminosis A is a result of consuming too much vitamin A. People with this condition can suffer from headaches, nausea, vomiting, hair loss, rashes, osteoporosis, and liver problems. Pregnant women should be careful not to consume too much vitamin A, since this can cause birth defects and miscarriages. Fortunately, a person would need to consume very large quantities of this vitamin (over 30,000 IU of vitamin A daily for more than a year) for the levels to become toxic. The recommended daily allowance (RDA) for vitamin A is 5,000 IU for men and 4,000 IU for women.

Vitamin C
Vitamin C has important functions in keeping us healthy. As an antioxidant, it works to remove dangerous free radicals that can cause cancer, heart disease, and stroke, and it benefits the heart by lowering cholesterol levels. It also aids the immune system in protecting against infection and heals wounds throughout the body.

Vitamin C plays a key role in the production of collagen, a substance that holds cells together. Collagen is found in bones, muscle, skin, and the eyes. In fact collagen is the major building block for many structures in the eye. For this reason, it is not surprising that people taking supplements containing vitamin C have been shown to have a reduced risk for cataracts. Since nearly the entire cornea and sclera are made up of collagen, vitamin C is sometimes prescribed to help the cornea heal from burns and other injuries. Fruits and vegetables are excellent sources of vitamin C (see page 119). However, consuming too much vitamin C (more than 2,000 mg/daily) is not recommended, since high doses can cause diarrhea and stomach upset.

Vitamin C deficiency can lead to a disease called scurvy. Scurvy was once common in sailors and pirates, who had little access to fresh fruits and vegetables during long voyages at sea. With this disease, people's muscles feel weak, their joints and muscles ache, they get a rash on their legs, and their gums bleed.

WAYS TO PREPARE FOODS TO RETAIN VITAMIN C
The process of preparing, cooking, or storing foods can lead to a loss of vitamin C. Ways to prevent the loss of vitamin C in your foods include:

- Eating raw fruits and vegetables quickly after buying them.
- Cutting vegetables just before cooking them.
- Using as little water as possible to cook foods that are rich in vitamin C.

Vitamin E

Vitamin E, an antioxidant, plays a key role in protecting the cells in the lens and the retina from damage. Studies have shown that this vitamin can delay the onset of cataracts and age-related macular degeneration and protect premature infants from retinal damage caused by exposure to too much oxygen early in life—a condition known as retinopathy of prematurity.

Vitamin E is found in a variety of food types and in many commercially available multivitamins. If you are considering taking vitamin E supplements, you should first check with your family doctor because vitamin E can thin the blood and interfere with certain medications. The tables on the next two pages provide a listing of the recommended daily allowance for each vitamin based on age, sex, and other factors (such as whether a person is pregnant or lactating).

Vitamin E supplements are best absorbed by the body when taken with a meal that contains some fat.

Carotenoids

There is truth behind the old adage that eating carrots is good for eyesight. This is because carrots are packed with beta carotene—a

FOODS HIGH IN VITAMINS A, C, AND E		
Vitamin A	Liver Cod-liver oil Egg yolk Milk Carrots Kale Collard greens	Sweet potato Spinach Apricot Melon Papaya Butter Cheese

Vitamin C	Citrus fruits
	Juices
	Strawberries
	Blueberries
	Cranberries
	Raspberries
	Watermelon
	Tomato
		Peppers
		  (green and red)
		Broccoli
		Cauliflower
		Cabbage
		Potato
		  (sweet and
		  white)

Vitamin E	Oils (including
	  vegetable, sunflower,
	  corn)
	Nuts
	Leafy vegetables
	Avocado
		Asparagus
		Whole milk
		Beef
		Turkey
		Soy
		Foods containing
		  whole grains

RECOMMENDED DAILY ALLOWANCES OF VITAMINS

Recommended daily allowances of each vitamin for different age groups.

Values in bold are recommended dietary allowances (RDAs); for all others, the adequate intakes (AIs) are shown, because RDAs are not available for those vitamins and age groups.

Compiled by the U.S. Department of Agriculture.

GROUP	Vitamin A (mcg)	Vitamin C (mg)	Vitamin D (mcg)	Vitamin E (mg)	Vitamin K (mcg)	Vitamin B6 (mg)	Vitamin B12 (mcg)
	RDA	RDA	AI	RDA	AI	RDA	RDA
INFANTS*							
0-6 months	400	40	5	4	2.0	0.1	0.4
7-12 months	500	50	5	5	2.5	0.3	0.5
CHILDREN							
1-3 years	**300**	**15**	5	**6**	30	**0.5**	**0.9**
4-8 years	**400**	**25**	5	**7**	55	**0.6**	**1.2**
MALES							
9-13 years	**600**	**45**	5	**11**	60	**1.0**	**1.8**
14-18 years	**900**	**65**	5	**15**	75	**1.3**	**2.4**
19-30 years	**900**	**75**	5	**15**	120	**1.3**	**2.4**
31-50 years	**900**	**75**	5	**15**	120	**1.3**	**2.4**
51-70 years	**900**	**75**	10	**15**	120	**1.7**	**2.4**
>70 years	**900**	**75**	15	**15**	120	**1.7**	**2.4**
FEMALES							
9-13 years	**600**	**45**	5	**11**	60	**1.0**	**1.8**
14-18 years	**700**	**65**	5	**15**	75	**1.2**	**2.4**
19-30 years	**700**	**75**	5	**15**	90	**1.3**	**2.4**
31-50 years	**700**	**75**	5	**15**	90	**1.3**	**2.4**
51-70 years	**700**	**75**	10	**15**	90	**1.5**	**2.4**
>70 years	**700**	**75**	15	**15**	90	**1.5**	**2.4**
PREGNANCY							
14-18 years	**750**	**80**	5	**15**	75	**1.9**	**2.6**
19-30 years	**770**	**85**	5	**15**	90	**1.9**	**2.6**
31-50 years	**770**	**85**	5	**15**	90	**1.9**	**2.6**
LACTATION							
14-18 years	**1,200**	**115**	5	**19**	75	**2.0**	**2.8**
19-30 years	**1,300**	**120**	5	**19**	90	**2.0**	**2.8**
31-50 years	**1,300**	**120**	5	**19**	90	**2.0**	**2.8**

*All the infant information is based upon AIs, since there is insufficient evidence to provide RDAs for infants.

Thiamin (mg)	Riboflavin (mg)	Niacin (mg)	Folate (mcg)	Pantothenic Acid (mg)	Biotin (mcg)	Choline (mg)
RDA	RDA	RDA	RDA	AI	AI	AI
0.2	0.3	2	65	1.7	5	125
0.3	0.4	4	85	1.8	6	150
0.5	0.5	6	150	2	8	200
0.6	0.6	8	200	3	12	250
0.9	0.9	12	300	4	20	375
1.2	1.3	16	400	5	25	550
1.2	1.3	16	400	5	30	550
1.2	1.3	16	400	5	30	550
1.2	1.3	16	400	5	30	500
1.2	1.3	16	400	5	30	500
0.9	0.9	12	300	4	20	375
1.0	1.0	14	400	5	25	400
1.1	1.1	14	400	5	30	425
1.1	1.1	14	400	5	30	425
1.1	1.1	14	400	5	30	425
1.1	1.1	14	400	5	30	425
1.4	1.4	18	600	6	30	450
1.4	1.4	18	600	6	30	450
1.4	1.4	18	600	6	30	450
1.4	1.6	17	500	7	35	550
1.4	1.6	17	500	7	35	550
1.4	1.6	17	500	7	35	550

substance found in various vegetables and other foods
that the body converts to vitamin A. This nourishes the
photoreceptors in the retina and may help protect the retina
against age-related macular degeneration.

Other carotenoids: lutein and zeaxanthin

Lutein and zeaxanthin are carotenoids that make up the
pigment in the macula, the central portion of the retina, which
is responsible for clear, central vision. These substances are
antioxidants that protect the eye against harmful, ultraviolet light
from the sun. Presently, a large study called AREDS II is assessing
whether taking these substances as supplements can help to
protect the eye against conditions such as macular degeneration and cataracts.

Zinc

The highest levels of the mineral zinc in the body are located in the retina.
The retinal pigment epithelium and choroid also contain high concentrations
of this mineral. In addition to its function as an antioxidant, zinc plays an
important role in helping the body absorb and process vitamin A. For these
reasons, researchers have been interested in learning whether supplements
that contain zinc may help protect the body against macular degeneration
and other eye diseases. In fact, a study compared two groups of patients
with macular degeneration. One was given 81 mg zinc supplements for
two years, and the other group did not receive supplementation with
this mineral. In this study, the group of patients who received the zinc
supplements experienced less vision loss as compared with the group that
did not receive the supplements. While the results of this study were quite
promising, other studies including
the large AREDS study showed no
association between supplementing the
body with zinc and the development
of macular degeneration. Additional
studies are needed to better understand
whether zinc supplements are useful in
protecting against diseases of the eye.

Oysters and other
shellfish are an excellent
source of zinc.

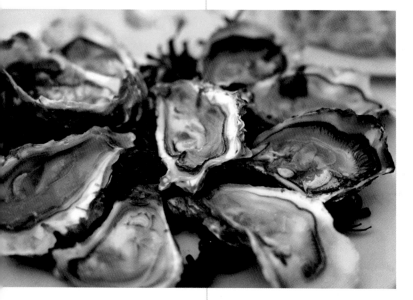

Docosahexaenoic acid (DHA)

Docosahexaenoic Acid (DHA) is
an omega-3-fatty acid found in oily
fish like tuna, mackerel, and salmon.
DHA and other polyuncarbonated
long chain fatty acids are present in
large quantities throughout the body,

especially in the brain and the photoreceptor cells of the retina. Studies have demonstrated that DHA can help protect against heart disease, reduce blood pressure and inflammation, and may help with depression. DHA has also plays a major role in the development of the brain and nervous system of neonates. There is currently a great deal of interest in whether omega-3-fatty acids can help protect against vision loss from macular degeneration. According to a recent study, eating foods containing high levels of DHA can cut in half a person's chances of getting the wet form of age-related macular degeneration. AREDS II—a large, ongoing clinical trial—will help eye-care professionals to learn more about the effects of DHA and other supplements on the health of the eye. Based on results from this study, eye-care professionals will be able to better advise patients on whether they should regularly take this supplement.

> Vegetarians and vegans generally have lower levels of DHA in their blood because foods of plant origin typically contain little, if any, DHA.

Natural treatments for dry eyes

Researchers have recently tested alpha-linolenic acid (ALA) in mice and found that eyedrops containing ALA helped protect the cornea from damage related to dry eyes. ALA is the parent compound of the family of omega-3 fatty acids. Flaxseed is the richest source of ALA, though various oils, nuts, and seeds also contain high levels of ALA. Studies are currently underway to determine whether this substance can help improve dry eyes in humans.

Herbal supplements for the eye

Although Chinese physicians have been using herbal products for hundreds of years, only recently have physicians and researchers in the Western world become interested in studying whether certain herbs or herbal supplements are beneficial to the human body. Two herbal supplements that are being investigated to determine whether they can improve the health of the eye are bilberry and Ginkgo biloba.

Bilberry *(Vaccinium myrtillus)* is a European shrub that produces berries similar to blueberries and huckleberries. These berries can be used to make jams and preserves. There are oral and eyedrop formulations containing bilberry. Researchers have been studying whether the high levels of antioxidants found in bilberry may improve eyesight. According to unsubstantiated anecdotal reports, World War

QUESTIONS TO ASK YOUR EYE DOCTOR

- Would any particular vitamins, minerals, or eye supplements be beneficial for my eyes?

- Based on my medical history and the medications I am taking for other health problems, are there certain vitamins, minerals, or eye supplements that may be harmful?

II pilots used bilberry to improve their night vision, although a relatively recent study by the U.S. Navy found that taking bilberry had no great effect on night vision. It has also been suggested that bilberry improves blood flow and reduces inflammation in the eye. A study using rats showed that bilberry may help prevent cataracts and macular degeneration. Unfortunately, however, no clinical trial in humans have tested bilberry's potential use in preventing, or treating any specific eye-related conditions.

Since bilberry and Ginkgo can interact with aspirin and products containing ibuprofen, resulting in thinning of the blood and excessive bleeding during surgery, it is important to let your physicians know if you are taking either of these supplements.

Ginkgo biloba is an herb that has been used in traditional Chinese medicine for centuries. Extracts from leaves of the ginkgo tree can be put into capsules, tablets, or herbal teas for consumption. Ginkgo biloba has been used to treat various medical conditions, including asthma, bronchitis, Alzheimer's disease, and sexual dysfunction. Ginkgo works by improving blood flow to the brain and other organs. Researchers have been studying whether taking Ginkgo may help treat patients with ocular conditions such as glaucoma and diabetic retinopathy. Recent studies have determined that in healthy individuals, Ginkgo supplements can, indeed, improve blood flow to the eye. Ongoing studies are assessing whether the use of this supplement can reduce the chances of worsening eye disease in patients with glaucoma.

If you are thinking of taking Ginkgo for your eyes, there are some important things you need to consider. First, since Ginkgo and other supplements are not regulated by institutions such as the U.S. Food and Drug Administration, the amount of Ginkgo can differ from one supplement to the next. Robert Abel, Jr., M.D., an ophthalmologist who is an authority

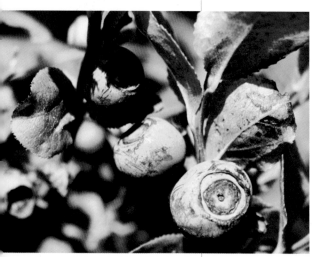

Bilberries look similar to blueberries. They commonly grow in Britain and other northern European countries.

CHINESE MEDICINE

Traditional Chinese medicine includes the use of dietary and herbal supplements, massage therapy, and acupuncture.

- Herbology is the Chinese method of combining medicinal herbs. Each mixture is tailored to the individual patient and his or her needs.

- Chinese massage therapy techniques focus on the energetics of the body. Manipulation techniques and acupressure points are used.

- Acupuncture points are situated on meridians (certain pathways in the body), along which *qi* (vital energy) flows.

using herbal supplements for eye-related problems, recommends checking to be sure your Ginkgo supplements contain at least 24 percent ginkgosides.

Alternative natural therapies

There are a number of natural remedies that claim to improve the health of the eye but have yet to be adequately tested by scientists to determine whether they are beneficial, have no effect, or are harmful to the eye.

Exercise and the eyes

Regular exercise is beneficial to the body in many ways. Studies have shown that exercise is good for the health of the heart and can reduce the chances of experiencing a stroke. Exercise has also been proven to help reduce blood pressure, lower cholesterol, and help reduce the risk of developing diabetes mellitus. Ongoing research is being conducted to determine whether exercising regularly is beneficial to the eye. One study found that people who exercised regularly had a 70 percent reduced likelihood of developing macular degeneration and other degenerative conditions of the eye. In this study, even those whose exercise consisted of walking regularly had a 30

UNPROVEN NATURAL SUPPLEMENTS		
Eyebright (*Euphrasia officinalis*)	This product has been used in folk medicine as a remedy for conjunctivitis, blepharitis, and other forms of surface irritations of the eye.	
Goldenseal (*Hydrastis Canadensis*)	Goldenseal is an herbal product that has been used by Native Americans to relieve sore, inflamed eyes.	
Pot marigold (*Calendula officinalis*)	This herbal remedy has been used to help with blepharitis, sties, and other conditions that cause eyelid inflammation.	
Vinpocetine (*from Vinca minor*)	Vinpocetine is a substance that is derived from the plant *Vinca minor*, a member of the periwinkle family. This herbal product has been used in Europe and Japan to treat cerebrovascular and cognitive disorders. It has been suggested that this remedy may improve blood flow to the eyes.	

percent reduced likelihood of developing macular degeneration. There is some evidence suggesting that aerobic exercise may protect the eye against glaucoma by lowering the pressure in the eye. Finally, since uncontrolled diabetes mellitus and high blood pressure can cause damage to various structures in the eye, regular exercise can protect against damage related to these conditions.

Toxins and the eyes

Smoking, the use of marijuana and alcohol are all known to have a negative impact upon our health. However, there are proven links between these toxins and the deterioration of the health of our eyes—from increasing the risk of cataracts to causing low eye pressure.

Smoking and the eyes

A great deal of evidence shows that cigarette smoke is harmful to one's health and increases the risk for early death. In fact, 15 percent of all deaths in the United States in a given year can be attributed to smoking. Cigarette smoking damages the lungs and the heart, and it has been strongly linked to multiple forms of cancer. Various structures in the eye can also be damaged by the 4,000 or so toxic ingredients found in tobacco smoke.

The two key ocular conditions linked to cigarette smoking are cataracts and age-related macular degeneration. In one study of more than 50,000 women, 45 to 67 years of age, those who smoked had a 63 percent increased risk of cataracts, compared with nonsmokers. Another study of over 22,000 men aged 40 to 84 found that those who smoked at least 20 cigarettes daily had more than double the risk of developing cataracts, compared with nonsmokers. A study from the United Kingdom showed that even people who used to be heavy smokers had a significantly elevated risk of developing cataracts. Not only does tobacco smoke increase the likelihood of developing cataracts, studies have shown that the progression of cataracts is also linked to cigarette smoking.

Age-related macular degeneration is another common cause of vision loss that has been linked to tobacco smoke. Since macular degeneration usually affects central vision, the visual impairment caused by this condition can be profound. Various large epidemiologic studies have shown that cigarette smokers are more than twice as likely as nonsmokers to develop age-related macular degeneration. While these studies showed that the risk of macular degeneration was reduced in people who quit smoking, even former smokers had a much higher risk of developing macular degeneration compared with nonsmokers. The fact that most

Smoking is the single most preventable cause of premature death in the United States.

forms of macular degeneration do not respond to treatment provides yet another reason to avoid cigarette smoking.

Both smokers themselves and people exposed frequently to second-hand smoke experience irritation to the conjunctiva as a result of the fumes and noxious chemicals in tobacco smoke. Eye-related symptoms of cigarette-smoke exposure include redness, stinging, burning, and tearing. Ongoing efforts to prohibit smoking in airplanes, restaurants, workplaces, and other indoor facilities should help reduce eye exposure to second-hand smoke.

Other eye conditions associated with cigarette smoke include anterior ischemic optic neuropathy (damage to the optic nerve from lack of blood flow), amaurosis fugax (temporary loss of sight due to a lack of blood flow to important structures in the eye), and strabismus (misalignment of the eyes) in children born to mothers who smoked during pregnancy.

Marijuana use and the eyes

Since the 1970s, eye care providers have been aware that a subset of people who smoke marijuana experience a temporary lowering of their eye pressure. Since elevated eye pressure is a known risk factor for glaucoma, there has been a great deal of interest in whether marijuana or some active ingredient in marijuana can be used to treat glaucoma. Studies have shown that smoking marijuana can lower eye pressure by up to 25 percent. While this pressure-lowering effect is as good as that produced by a number of commonly prescribed anti-glaucoma eyedrops, there are several reasons why the Institute of Medicine, the National Eye Institute, the American Academy of Ophthalmology, the American Medical Association, and most eye care professionals advise against the use of marijuana to treat glaucoma. First, smoking marijuana is a poor treatment option because the eye-pressure–lowering effect lasts only 3–4 hours. So, for patients to achieve sustained pressure reduction from this herbal drug, they would need to smoke 7–8 times daily. Second, high doses of marijuana are needed to get these pressure-lowering benefits. Since smoking marijuana causes cognitive impairment and various other side effects, including lung damage, many eye care professionals feel that the risks of exposure to this drug outweigh the potential benefit, especially given that various safe and effective medical and surgical treatments for glaucoma are currently available. Researchers are trying to identify the specific substances in marijuana responsible for the pressure-lowering effects on the eye. Once these

Other effects of marijuana on the eye include conjunctival hyperemia (redness), dryness of the eyes, double vision, sensitivity to light, and the reduced ability to focus clearly on objects up close.

substances have been identified, researchers may be able to develop new drugs for glaucoma that can lower the eye pressure without subjecting patients to the toxic side effects of this drug.

Alcohol and the eyes

Alcohol is known to affect the eyes in a variety of ways. When an individual is acutely intoxicated, the eyes appear bloodshot, the pupils can be larger than normal, it can be difficult to adjust to bright lights, and vision can be distorted. In addition, a person who is under the influence of alcohol often has difficulty with tasks that involve hand-eye coordination. Studies have also revealed that alcohol also affects the ability of people to follow objects as they go across their field of vision. Since hand-eye coordination and the tracking of objects is particularly important when operating a motor vehicle, these studies reinforce the dangers of driving while intoxicated. Long-term use of alcohol can damage the liver, which can, in turn, lead to the build-up of wastes in the body, a condition known as jaundice. People who are jaundiced have yellowing of their skin and yellowing of the whites of their eyes.

Alcohol consumption during pregnancy increases the risk of giving birth to a child with fetal alcohol syndrome. This syndrome is characterized by low birth weight, developmental delay, abnormal appearance of the face and eyes, learning difficulties, and abnormalities of other organs. Children with fetal alcohol syndrome are more likely to have weaker than normal vision, strabismus (misalignment of the eyes), and cataracts early in life.

While excessive use of alcohol can lead to damage to the eyes, as outlined above, researchers are presently studying whether a compound called resveratrol, which is found in red wine, may actually be beneficial for the health of the eye. Resveratrol is an antioxidant that is present in the skin of red grapes. Some studies have found that this compound may help protect people from developing heart disease. Ongoing studies are being conducted to determine whether resveratrol can protect against other diseases associated with aging. In the eye, studies using this compound in rats showed that resveratrol may be protective against the formation of cataracts. It is unknown whether resveratrol or the moderate consumption of red wine that contains resveratrol can prevent cataracts or other eye diseases in humans, though researchers are presently conducting studies to learn more about the effects of resveratrol on the eye.

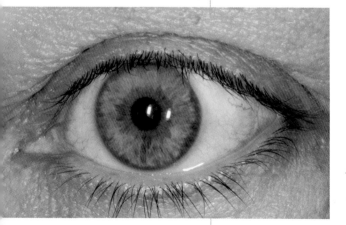

Liver damage from alcohol abuse can lead to jaundice. A prominent sign of jaundice is the yellow discoloration of the conjunctiva (the whites of the eyes).

Supplement summary

Many of the supplements we explore in this chapter have not yet been proven in clinical trials to benefit the eye and further research is needed before we know for sure whether they are effective at preventing and/or reducing vision loss. Moreover, it is important to be aware that these herbal products are not regulated by the FDA and that some of them have side effects (such as increasing the risk of bleeding during eye surgery which can be very serious and result in permanent blindness). You must always consult with your eye professional before using these products.

OPTICAL ILLUSION

In many countries including the United States, medications require extensive testing to determine that they are safe and effective before they can be marketed and sold to consumers. However, vigorous testing is not required for vitamins and dietary supplements.

NATURAL SUPPLEMENTS

Supplement	Function	Side effects
Vitamin A	Aids the production of tears. Supports the rods in the retina.	High in saturated fat and cholesterol – excessive amounts can be harmful.
Vitamin C	Helps lower cholesterol levels. Supports the immune system. Produces collagen.	Consuming too much (over 2,000 mg/ daily) can cause stomach upset.
Vitamin E	Protects lens cells and the retina from damage.	Can act as a blood thinner and affect medications.
Carotenoids	Provide nourishment to photoreceptors in the retina.	Too much beta-carotene can turn the color of skin to yellow or orange.
Zinc	Helps the body to absorb and process vitamin A. May protect against macular degeneration.	A zinc dose of 40 mg is approved safe to use by FDA and a zinc dosage more than this can pose certain risks.
DHA	Help reduce chances of vision loss from age-related macular degeneration.	Nausea, gas and a fishy aftertaste.
Bilberry	May help to improve vision. Enhances blood flow and reduces inflammation in the eye.	Mild digestive distress, skin rashes and drowsiness. Can also interfere with aspirin.
Ginkgo biloba	Improves blood flow to the eye and may help ocular conditions such as glaucoma and diabetic retinopathy.	Can cause headaches, a bad temper, anxiety, diarrhea and nausea.

7

Cosmetic Eye Care

Our eyes hold the key to our facial expressions. Because of this, many of us feel that the appearance of our eyes is an extremely important part of our self-image. While natural aging affects the appearance of your eyes, along with the rest of your body, you can target these changes to slow down or reverse the signs of aging and make your eyes appear more youthful and refreshed.

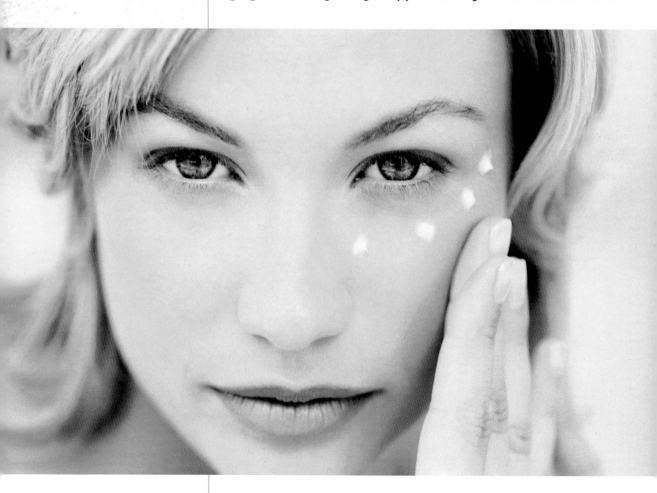

Eye cosmetics

The simplest way to change the appearance of your eyes is to use eye cosmetics. Eyelid pigments have been used throughout history for cosmetic reasons—and they were also used as early as 4000 B.C.E. to treat eye infections.

Because the skin of your eyelids is exceedingly thin, eye cosmetics are formulated to be non-irritating to this sensitive area. In case cosmetics have accidental contact with your eyeball, it is important that manufacturers also test their eye cosmetics. You will find that many eye cosmetics are labeled as "hypoallergenic," "ophthalmologist tested," "allergy tested," "safe for sensitive skin," and so on, yet cosmetic companies are not required to perform any standardized safety testing. In the United States, for instance, the Food and Drug Administration prohibits cosmetic companies from using known harmful chemicals and allows only certain coloring chemicals to be used in eye shadows, but states that cosmetic companies are responsible for the safety of their products and ingredients before marketing them.

For sensitive souls

The thin skin of your eyelid is one of the areas of your body most prone to irritation and allergy, also known as contact dermatitis. However, since we all have different types and levels of sensitivities, it's wise to test all the new cosmetics you buy before you apply them to the skin around your eyes.

- Keep in mind that many sponge applicators sold with eye shadows contain latex, which is a source of allergy for some people.
- Eyelid cosmetic removal products can irritate the skin of sensitive individuals. For this reason, you should avoid waterproof eye cosmetics that are difficult to remove with just water if you have especially sensitive eyelid skin.

COMMON COSMETIC INGREDIENTS THAT CAN CAUSE EYELID CONTACT DERMATITIS

If you have a history of this type of allergy, you might find it helpful to avoid the ingredients listed below.

- Preservatives: parabens, phenyl mercuric acetate, imidazolidinyl urea, quaternium-15, potassium sorbate
- Antioxidants: butylated hydroxyanisole, butylated hydroxytoluene, di-tert-butyl-hydroquinone
- Resins: colophony
- Pearlescent additives: bismuth oxychloride
- Emollients: lanolin, propylene glycol
- Fragrances
- Pigment contaminants: nickel

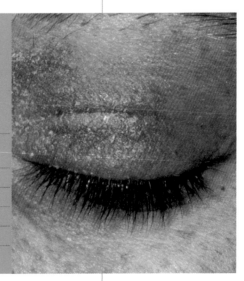

• If you wear contact lenses, you should insert them before applying eye cosmetics and take them out before cosmetic removal.

Contact dermatitis that appears to be related to cosmetics can sometimes be a sign of other underlying skin or eye problems. If you suspect your contact dermatitis is related to your cosmetics, but the redness, irritation, or swelling doesn't go away when you stop using them, be sure to see your eye doctor or dermatologist to determine if there is another cause.

Choosing cosmetics for sensitive skin is an important part of eye care. Some dermatologists suggest that, even if you are prone to contact dermatitis, there are still some ways to minimize your risk of skin irritation while using cosmetics to enhance your appearance. Whenever possible, choose powder cosmetics over creams or lotions since these tend to be less irritating to sensitive skin. Avoid waterproof cosmetics, since these take more effort to remove and contain more ingredients that can be irritating compared to water-soluble makeup. Since bacteria can contaminate cosmetics, especially if they are old, be sure to purchase fresh cosmetics on a regular basis.

Eyeliner and mascara, which are the cosmetics usually used closest to the eye, should be replaced every three months. Choosing these cosmetics in the color black can help since other color pigments can be more irritating. It is advisable to use eyeliners and eyebrow makeup in pencil forms, or apply powder eye shadows gently with an eyeliner brush to avoid creams close to the eye. While deep, vibrant colors of eye shadow can look glamorous, these brightly colored pigments can irritate the skin, so stick with neutral or earth-toned shadows. Choose matte eye shadows rather than frosted, iridescent, or shiny types, since the ingredients that add the sparkle can also cause skin flare-ups.

In general, it may help to avoid cosmetics with more than 10 ingredients listed, since more ingredients can mean more chance of skin irritation. For those with very sensitive skin, select cosmetics without chemical sunscreens, especially near the eye area. Avoid wearing nail polish, since the strong chemicals in polish can irritate your skin, especially when your nails touch your face. Facial foundations should be cream or powder formulations for the least irritation; if you choose a liquid foundation, it should be based on silicone derivatives, such as cyclomethicone or dimethicone.

Mascara

You can use mascara to accentuate your eyelashes and make your eyes appear larger; mascara is most commonly sold in liquid form and comes in water-based and waterproof types. Water-soluble types of mascara can be less irritating than waterproof types, and removing water-soluble mascara is less irritating for the skin of your eyelids. However, water-soluble mascara is more prone to bacterial contamination, so you'll tend to find more preservatives have been added than you'll find in waterproof mascara. Even though manufacturers add these chemicals to reduce the risk of bacterial infections, it's still advisable to replace your mascara tube frequently and avoid sharing it with other people.

Mascara is less commonly available in cake form, which is the least irritating type if you have especially sensitive eyelid skin, or in single-use tubes, which can be a good option if you are prone to bacterial infections. Applying several coats of mascara to just the tips of your lashes, rather than to their entire length, is another strategy for minimizing the amount of mascara that comes in contact with your eyelids or eyeball.

> You should replace your mascara and liquid eyeliner tubes three months after they have been opened.

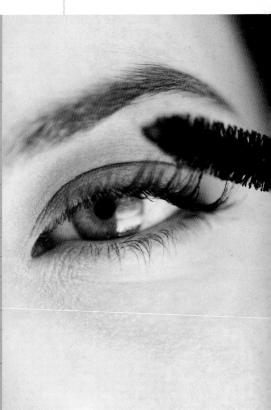

SAFETY TIPS

- **Wash your hands before applying makeup to avoid transferring bacteria to your eye.**
- **Keep your makeup applicators clean.**
- **Don't keep your cosmetics in extreme temperatures (such as in a hot car) since the preservatives may break down, allowing bacteria to grow.**
- **Bacteria may grow more easily in "natural" or "preservative-free" cosmetics.**
- **Don't moisten eye cosmetics with water or saliva, since bacteria grow well in moist environments.**
- **Don't share makeup or makeup applicators with others.**
- **Avoid applying makeup while driving or riding in a vehicle.**
- **Remove your makeup before going to sleep each night.**
- **Don't use a pin or other sharp, pointed object to separate your eyelashes.**
- **Don't apply makeup to broken or irritated skin.**
- **If you experience severe, prolonged eye pain, see an eye doctor right away.**
- **If you develop an eye infection, stop using eye makeup. Discard and replace your eye makeup after the infection has gone away.**

Eyeliner

Eyeliner, which can make your eyes appear larger and more well-defined, is commonly available in liquid and pencil forms. The liquid types are as prone to bacterial contamination as mascara, while pencil eyeliners are generally less irritating and easier to apply, and sharpening the pencil reduces any previous contamination of the tip. Avoid applying any eyeliner inside the lash line, since this can inadvertently injure your eyeball and irritate the delicate tissues of your conjunctiva and cornea.

If you're considering permanent makeup, remember that permanent means exactly that. While many types of tattoo ink can be removed with laser treatments, it can take numerous laser treatments to achieve a satisfactory result.

Permanent makeup

Permanent makeup has been growing in popularity in recent years. Eyeliner and eyebrow tattoos in particular can save you the trouble of having to use cosmetics regularly. Bear in mind that, while the inks used are subject to government regulation, they have not been approved for injection into the skin, and there are no set government regulations governing the actual practice of tattooing.

While permanent makeup can be a boon, especially if you have trouble applying cosmetics because of physical difficulties, you should understand the risks and benefits of these procedures. It's best to be sure that the person performing your procedure is experienced and that his equipment is sterile. There are rare reports of scarring and skin allergy to tattoo dyes, and there is a very small risk of bacterial infection.

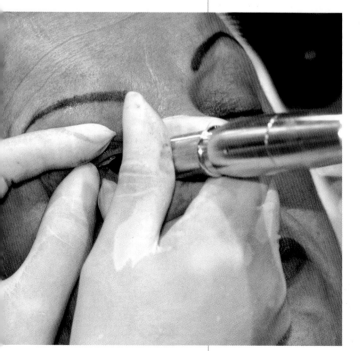

Permanent eyeliner being applied.

Anti-aging cosmetics

While a myriad of eye creams and lotions are available on the market, in general they won't dramatically improve your appearance. Creams and lotions can help to moisturize the delicate skin of your eyelids, which can marginally help the appearance of lines and wrinkles, but these effects are minimal and temporary. Like other eye cosmetics, eyelid creams and lotions are not subject to strict government regulations, and the anti-aging claims made by their manufacturers aren't required to be tested or proven. However, most eyelid creams and lotions are unlikely to cause harm as long as they do not irritate your eyes or your eyelid skin. If they do irritate, be sure to stop using them since repeated usage is likely to make your discomfort worse.

Anti-aging eyelid treatments

With the popularity of cosmetic eye treatments exploding in recent years, it can be useful to understand what treatments are available and how they might work for you.

Protecting your eyelids from the sun

While medical research has shown that retinoic acid and sunscreen agents decrease facial wrinkles in general, using such strong chemicals on the thin skin of your eyelids can potentially irritate your eyes. We know that ultraviolet light from the sun causes much of the aging damage to the skin of our eyelids, and sun exposure is something that we can all control. Not only will you be taking a step to preserve the youthful appearance of your eyes, but you'll also be reducing your risk of skin cancer, which can affect your eyelids as well. And, as an added benefit, shielding your eyes from sunlight throughout your life can lessen your chances of developing cataracts and macular degeneration.

OPTICAL ILLUSION

Cosmetic companies make loud claims about the miracle-working, anti-aging effects of their eye creams and lotions, but generally these creams have only minimal and temporary effects on lines and wrinkles.

Puffy eyelids

Have you ever noticed that your eyelids are sometimes puffy? This puffiness happens when the thin skin of your eyelids shows signs of swelling of your eyelid tissues under the skin. Many people wake up with puffy eyelids because as you lie flat, excess fluid accumulates in your eyelid tissues when you sleep. This type of puffiness usually goes away quickly after you wake up and remain upright, letting gravity help the extra fluid to drain away from your head. Consuming too much salt, caffeine, or alcohol can contribute to eyelid puffiness, so if this is a problem for you, try to avoid these substances. Get plenty of rest, since sleep deprivation can cause this puffiness as well.

Other reasons to have puffy eyelids include aging as well as more serious medical problems. As we get older, our thin eyelid skin stretches and becomes looser, allowing the natural fat pads under the skin to bulge forward. This type of puffiness doesn't fluctuate throughout the day and is best treated by surgery if desired (see "blepharoplasty" section on page 139). While pregnancy and hormonal changes can cause eyelid puffiness that comes and goes, more serious problems, such as contact dermatitis, allergies, thyroid eye disease, and other medical problems can cause more severe eyelid puffiness. If you are concerned that your eyelid puffiness doesn't go away and is not merely from aging, see your eye doctor.

Wearing sunglasses with ultraviolet protection or a hat to shield your eyes and eyelids from the sun is the best way to prevent sun damage to the delicate skin of your eyelids.

Avoid putting hemorrhoid cream, cucumbers, or tea bags on your eyes, as these can irritate your eyeballs. Cool compresses are a safer way to relieve temporary eyelid puffiness.

To help eyelid puffiness go away, try using cool compresses. To do this, wring a clean washcloth out in cool water, close your eyes, and put this compress on your closed eyelids for five minutes.

Dark under-eye circles

Nearly everyone has noticed dark under-eye circles in themselves or in someone they know. These dark circles can make us look older or more tired. Our genes have a lot to do with whether we are prone to developing these dark circles, which appear when our thin lower eyelid skin contains more pigment than the rest of our facial skin or when the darker blood vessels under this skin show through. Aging, since it causes our eyelid skin to thin over time, can also make dark circles more apparent.

While we can't change the genes we were born with or slow the passage of time, we can avoid sun exposure and wear sunglasses, since sunlight can worsen these dark circles. People with allergies may be prone to developing dark circles, so avoiding allergens or treating allergies with antihistamines can help in these cases. More aggressive treatment options include injecting cosmetic fillers to plump up the under-eye area, or laser skin resurfacing of the lower eyelid skin (see "Cosmetic Facial Fillers" and "Laser Skin Resurfacing" sections below).

Botox

Botox is the most popular cosmetic medical treatment in North America today. Botox is a medicine that weakens the muscles of your face, resulting in fewer lines and wrinkles. Botox is injected with a tiny needle into the facial muscles right underneath your skin. Botox is made from a naturally occurring substance that causes muscle weakness in small doses and muscle paralysis in larger doses. It is generally safe if injected properly and has other medical uses besides cosmetic treatments, such as relaxing muscles in your eyelids or cheeks that cause unwanted facial spasms.

Botox can be useful for softening crow's feet (the wrinkles at the outside corners of your eyes), the frown lines between the eyebrows, horizontal forehead

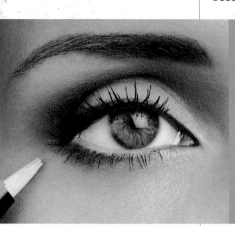

DARK CIRCLE CREAMS

The multitude of cosmetic eyelid creams on the market that are targeted for dark circles generally hasn't been shown to have major effects in research studies. Using a cosmetic concealer is perhaps the simplest way to cover up dark under-eye circles to make you look more youthful and refreshed.

lines, and vertical lip lines, and for shaping the action and height of your eyebrows. The injections generally take a few minutes, and you'll see the softening effects within several days. You don't need any special preparation for the injections, and you can return to your regular activities immediately afterward. Once the effect of the medication has worn off, Botox can be injected again if you wish.

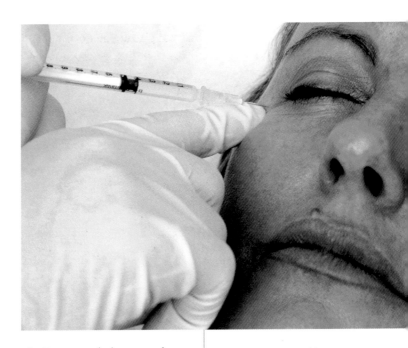

If you're planning to undergo Botox treatments, look for a doctor who has experience performing this type of procedure. There can sometimes be mild side effects, such as weakness of a nearby muscle that could cause facial asymmetry or a droopy eyelid or lip, for example. Fortunately because the effects of Botox are not permanent, any unwanted muscle weakness usually also disappears with time.

Botox being injected in the crow's feet area.

To avoid spreading Botox to a nearby muscle, it's best to avoid touching the area of your face that was injected for several hours after the treatment. You may experience mild discomfort from the injections along with a tiny amount of bruising, which generally fades quickly. The risk of infection is minimal with the standard use of sterile needles.

Cosmetic facial fillers

If you'd like to reduce the appearance of facial wrinkles, you may also want to consider cosmetic soft tissue fillers. These are injected under your skin to fill a wrinkle and make your skin appear plumper and fuller in that area. In particular, frown lines between the eyebrows, wrinkles around the lips, and creases along the sides of the nose and mouth and around the lips can be softened by these facial fillers, giving you a more youthful appearance. Scars or other unwanted dimples in the skin can also be made less obvious with facial fillers. Cosmetic soft tissue filler treatments are sometimes performed alongside Botox treatments, since these two types of treatments can complement one another. Botox softens wrinkles by targeting the muscles of the face, while cosmetic facial fillers fill and soften areas of lost volume under the skin due to age.

There are several substances commonly used as facial fillers:

- Hyaluronic acid is a flexible substance that occurs naturally in your skin and is manufactured in an injectable form. Available brands of hyaluronic

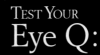

TEST YOUR
Eye Q:

True or False?
Botox is made from botulinum toxin, a substance that can be dangerous in large doses but is harmless in the small amounts used for this cosmetic treatment.
True

acid include Restylane, Perlane, Juvederm, and Hylaform. The effects of hyaluronic acid typically last for 6–12 months before an injection may need to be repeated.

- Collagen is another injectable substance that is normally made by your body's natural tissues. Collagen injections last for somewhat less time than hyaluronic acid injections.
- Synthetic microspheres (such as Radiesse) are another choice for these treatments, and the effects of this substance last longer than hyaluronic acid.

Advances in technology have made the effects of cosmetic soft tissue fillers more natural and attractive than ever before. The risks of treatment are mild, but include the rare possibility of infection as well as mild bruising after the injections that will fade with time. Some physicians numb the area with anesthetic cream, anesthetic injections, or ice, and then the filler is injected with a tiny needle into the area of the wrinkle.

COSMETIC FACIAL FILLERS

Substance	Brand name examples	What is it?	Typical usage	Length of effectiveness
Hyaluronic acid	Restylane Perlane Juvederm Hylaform	Hyaluronic acid is a flexible substance naturally found in the skin	Plumping lips; filling facial creases, wrinkles, and hollow scars	6 to 12 months
Collagen	Cosmoderm Cosmoplast	Collagen is a natural protein found in the skin	Filling facial lines and wrinkles	2 to 4 months
Synthetic microspheres	Radiesse, Artefill	Calcium hydro-xylapatite (a mineral found in bone) or PMMA (a synthetic material) microspheres are suspended in a water-based gel	Filling deep facial folds and creases, especially smile lines	6 months or longer
Fat	Not applicable	Your own fat is removed by liposuction from elsewhere in your body and used as a facial filler	Filling facial folds, enhancing facial fullness and contours	Variable

You'll see the effects of the treatment immediately, and you may have mild swelling for the first 24 hours. You don't need any special preparation for the treatment, and you can return to your usual activities afterward. As with Botox, if you are considering these types of treatments, be sure to see a physician who has experience with the cosmetic aspects of the face and who takes the time to understand your wishes and expectations.

Cosmetic eye surgery

Cosmetic eye surgery may be the best way to address many of the more obvious signs that your eyes are aging. These surgeries have the potential to help you feel better about your appearance and yourself. Make sure that you're aware of the costs of the procedure in advance, since cosmetic procedures typically are not covered by medical insurance, so you will most likely be required to pay out-of-pocket for these surgeries.

Blepharoplasty

Have you ever wondered if saggy eyelid skin can be made to look smoother and younger? As we age, the smooth, thin skin of our upper and lower eyelids becomes more saggy and loose. The underlying muscles of your eyelids also stretch over time so that the natural fat behind your eyelids can bulge forward, resulting in sagging upper eyelids and bags under your eyes. These aging changes can make you look older and more tired and can even alter your facial expressions. Excess sagging of the upper eyelid skin, if severe enough, can also obscure your upward peripheral vision. Sun exposure and your genes also contribute to this aging change of the eyelids. Blepharoplasty is a term that means surgery to improve the look of your eyelids.

Upper lid blepharoplasty involves your surgeon making a small incision that is hidden in the natural crease of your upper eyelid. Excess skin, muscle, and possibly fat will then be removed from your upper eyelid. The incision is closed with tiny stitches, which are normally removed in 1–2 weeks. If your upper eyelid is also droopy, a ptosis repair can be performed during surgery through the same incision.

Lower lid blepharoplasty can help improve the appearance of your eyes if your lower eyelids are droopy or you have bags under your eyes. Lower lid blepharoplasty can be performed from the inside of your lower eyelid (the side against the eyeball) to remove bulging fat that causes bags, or from the outside of your eyelid to remove excess fat and skin. If done from the outside, tiny stitches will be needed to close the incision, which is located just under

OPTICAL ILLUSION
While the different types of cosmetic facial fillers may sound similar, certain fillers are better for specific types of lines and wrinkles than others. Let your doctor help you choose which filler is appropriate for you.

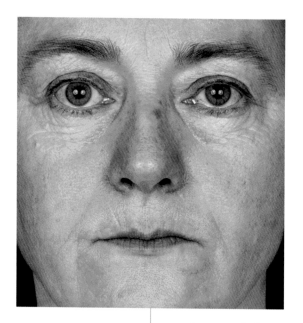

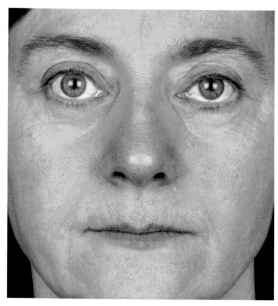

TOP LEFT Before upper lid blepharoplasty.

TOP RIGHT After upper lid blepharoplasty. Note the decreased fullness of the upper eyelids.

your lower eyelashes. Sometimes removing the bags, or bulging fat, from the lower eyelids results in baggy skin once the fat is gone. This saggy skin can be smoothed and tightened with laser skin resurfacing or a chemical peel afterward.

Blepharoplasty is an outpatient procedure that can be performed in your surgeon's office, surgery center, or hospital. Whether your surgeon performs upper lid blepharoplasty, lower lid blepharoplasty, or both upper and lower lid blepharoplasty together depends on your individual cosmetic needs, but both right and left sides typically undergo the procedure during the same surgery. You might be given mild oral or intravenous sedation while the procedure is performed under local anesthetic. Mild bruising and swelling are common after surgery, and typically fade away with time. Your surgeon may ask you to use ice packs and antibiotic ointment on your stitches as your incisions heal. As with any surgery, risks of significant bleeding, scarring, vision loss, and infection are possible, though rare. Under- or over-correction can also occur with blepharoplasty. Be sure to find a surgeon with whom you are comfortable and who listens to you, so you have the best chance of being satisfied with your results.

You should tell your surgeon before the procedure if you take any blood thinners, have bleeding problems, or have problems with dry eyes.

Droopy eyelid repair

When your upper lid droops, the medical term for this is ptosis. In adults, ptosis is most commonly a result of aging, but it can also be caused by injury or by muscular or neurologic diseases. Ptosis can occur rarely in infants, and in this situation it is usually caused by abnormal development of the eyelid muscle (called the levator) that opens the eyelid.

In the type of adult ptosis that is caused by aging, the tendon that attaches the levator muscle to your eyelid becomes stretched over time so that your eyelid droops.

If one or both of your upper eyelids droops, you may notice that it's difficult to open your eyes fully, or that your eyebrows ache from rising to open your eyes wider, compensating for your droopy eyelids. You may experience eye fatigue, especially when you're reading. You may even notice that you see and feel better if you lift your eyelids with your own finger. Ptosis generally requires repair if your peripheral vision is significantly blocked by your droopy upper lid (the lid covers much of your pupil), but it can also be repaired for cosmetic reasons if it is milder and covers less of your pupil.

It's important to see an eye doctor with experience in eyelid surgery if you want to have your ptosis corrected with surgery. Your eye doctor should rule out other causes of droopy eyelids besides aging, because certain muscle or nerve diseases that can cause ptosis have different treatments from the type of surgery performed for age-related ptosis. The goal of surgery is to raise your upper eyelid so it doesn't block your peripheral vision and to achieve a symmetric result with your other upper eyelid. If you have an abnormal levator muscle, however, it may be difficult to achieve a completely normal eyelid position and function after surgery.

Ptosis surgery is an outpatient surgery that can be performed in your surgeon's office, surgery center, or hospital, depending on your surgical needs. Most adults are given a mild sedative, either by mouth or intravenously, and then the procedure is performed under local anesthetic. If both of your upper eyelids need surgery, your surgeon will probably operate on both of them during the same procedure. Some surgeons judge the position of the eyelids while they are operating by asking you to open and close your eyes during the procedure. You'll have stitches after the surgery,

LEFT Marking the incision in ptosis surgery.
RIGHT Closing the incision with stitches.

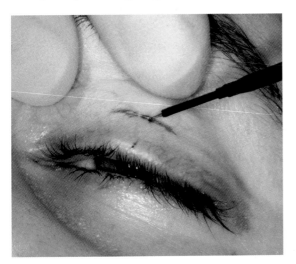

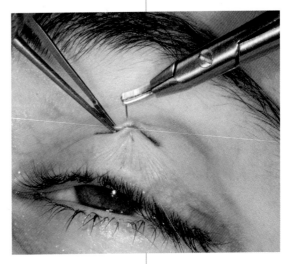

which your surgeon may remove one to two weeks later. You can also expect mild bruising and swelling after the surgery, which normally goes away in one to two weeks as well. Your surgeon may recommend that you use ice packs and antibiotic ointment on your stitches during the healing period.

As with every surgery, there are risks with ptosis repair. Significant bleeding, scarring, and infection are possible, but rather uncommon. Remember to tell your surgeon before the procedure if you take any blood thinners or have bleeding problems. Overcorrecting by lifting the lid too high, thus causing dry eyes, or not achieving a symmetric result are also possible. In some situations, your surgeon may have to perform a touch-up or corrective procedure to improve any asymmetry or overcorrection that persists after your swelling has gone away.

QUESTIONS TO ASK YOUR EYE DOCTOR

• Would my surgery just be for cosmetic purposes? Or, do my eyelids droop enough that the surgery is considered medically necessary because my eyelids block my vision?

• What side effects will I experience after the procedure?

Brow lift

If you've developed a sagging brow or forehead over time and feel that this makes you look older or more tired, you may want to know more about brow or forehead lifts. In this type of surgery, the skin and muscles of the forehead are lifted to provide a younger, smoother appearance. Some people's brows droop so much that their upper eyelids look droopy as well; a brow lift can also help in this situation. The final result of a brow lift is a smoother forehead, repositioned eyebrows, and reduced fullness at the base of the nose. These changes can make you look younger, refreshed, and more relaxed.

Endoscopic brow lifts are also known as forehead lifts. Brow lifts can be performed with incisions above both eyebrows, but this tends to leave visible scars. Endoscopic brow lifts are more commonly performed for cosmetic purposes. In this surgery, small incisions are made in your hairline, where they will ultimately be almost invisible. A very small camera and endoscopic instruments are then inserted though the incisions to perform the surgery under the skin and muscles of your forehead. Once lifted, the tissues are secured in place with dissolvable devices.

Brow lifts are performed as outpatient surgery and, just as with other types of cosmetic surgery, have small risks of

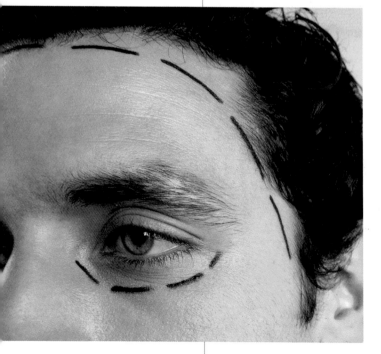

Areas to be targeted in brow lift surgery and lower lid blepharoplasty.

significant bleeding, scarring, facial numbness, and infection. Your typical recovery time will be up to several weeks. Tell your surgeon prior to surgery about any blood thinners you take or any bleeding problems you may have. To make sure you are completely satisfied with the results you get, it's important to communicate with your surgeon about your desires and expectations before surgery to help you decide if this procedure is right for you.

Repair of eyelids that turn in or out

Aging can make some people's upper or lower eyelids turn in or out, which results in a poor eyelid position. "Ectropion" is the term for when your eyelids turn out, while "entropion" describes when your eyelids turn in. Either can occur as the muscles and tendons that hold your eyelids in place against the eyeball loosen with age, and the eyelids lose their elasticity and normal position. As a result, your eyelids can no longer perform their job of protecting and lubricating your eyeball as well as they could before. Ectropion and entropion can lead to a poor cosmetic appearance or, even more important, can result in irritation or significant dryness to the eyeball. If the eyelids turn out, they can't hold your eye's normal tears against your eyeball to lubricate it properly, and your eye may feel irritated and dry as a result. In entropion, your eyelashes can point inward toward your eyeball, which causes rubbing and constant irritation to the eye's surface.

While most cases of eyelids turning in or out are due to aging, there are other causes that your eye doctor should eliminate. In some cases, paralysis of the facial nerve that controls the eyelid muscles can lead to an eyelid turning out. Skin allergies or scarring from skin diseases, chemical burns, or prior surgery can also cause these eyelid problems. It is important to know why your eyelid is poorly positioned, because different causes may require different sorts of treatments.

Procedures to correct turned eyelids are commonly performed if the cause is aging. As with other eyelid surgeries, these repairs are outpatient procedures, performed with local anesthetic and possibly some oral or intravenous sedation. If both your eyes have the same type of eyelid problem, both eyes will undergo surgery at the same time. Depending on the type of repair, you may have stitches that your surgeon will remove one to two weeks after surgery. Some bruising and swelling should be expected as you heal, and you may be asked to use ice packs and antibiotic ointment during that time.

The risks of repairing eyelids that turn in or out are fairly small, but include significant bleeding, scarring, infection, or the possibility that the repair may have to be repeated or touched up in the future if the results do not last long-term. Surgery to fix this type of eyelid problem helps

True or False?

Eyelids that turn in or turn out are just a cosmetic problem.

False

Having eyelids that turn in or out can cause problems with your eye health by making the surface of your eyeball dry or irritated.

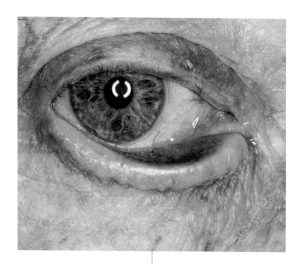

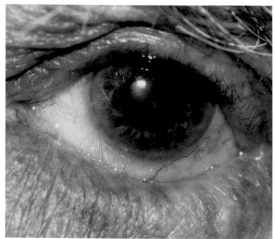

most people, especially since turned eyelids not only can look cosmetically unacceptable but can also negatively affect the health of your eyes.

Laser skin resurfacing around the eyes

Have you ever wondered if there's a procedure out there that can improve wrinkled facial skin? Do you have skin that has other signs of aging or damage, such as irregular pigmentation? If so, you may want to know more about laser skin resurfacing, which is becoming increasingly popular. The outermost layers of the skin are vaporized with a carbon dioxide or Erbium laser and the laser energy also causes the underlying collagen in the skin to tighten. As your skin heals, new healthy skin cells grow to replace the top layer, which can reduce the appearance of fine lines and improve your skin's texture.

You can target certain areas of your face with laser skin resurfacing by itself, or the procedure can be combined with other surgeries. For instance, in lower eyelid blepharoplasty, after the excess saggy muscle tissue and bulging fat are removed from the lower lids, the excess skin of your lower eyelids may be looser than desired. Laser skin resurfacing can then be performed to tighten this skin and improve your appearance.

Avoid excessive sun exposure and use sunscreen generously for up to a year after your laser skin resurfacing, as sunlight can cause irregular pigmentation of the treated skin.

Before you decide whether laser skin resurfacing is right for you, make sure to find a doctor who has experience in this area and who will take the time to talk to you, answer your questions, and discuss your goals. Laser skin resurfacing can greatly improve the look of your skin, but it is not appropriate for all types of aging changes. Also, because aging is a continuous process, the results of this procedure are not usually permanent. Your doctor should help you decide if your particular skin needs are best served by laser skin resurfacing.

Laser skin resurfacing is an outpatient procedure, typically performed in your doctor's office, in an outpatient surgery center, or in a hospital. It's usually performed with local anesthetics and possibly oral or intravenous sedation. It takes time for your new skin cells to grow back after the resurfacing is performed, so swelling and crusting are common after the treatment, and you should expect your skin to look red or pink for up to several weeks. Your doctor may ask you to use ointment on your face or give you other instructions to follow as your skin heals. The risks are small but include irregular skin pigmentation or texture, infection, or scarring. Carefully shielding your skin from the sun will help protect your new, smoother skin from further aging changes caused by ultraviolet light as time goes on.

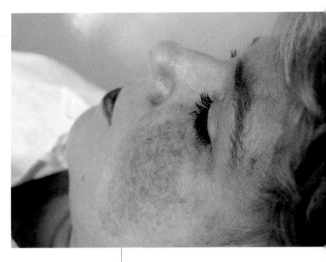

Laser skin resurfacing and chemical peels will result in temporary redness of the treated skin during the healing period.

Chemical peels around the eyes

Our skin is constantly shedding its outermost layers and replacing them with newer skin cells from deeper down in the skin. As we get older, this turnover of our skin slows down, leaving us with older, sun-damaged top layers of skin that remain and can contribute to fine lines, wrinkles, and an older appearance. Another way to rejuvenate your skin, besides laser skin resurfacing, is by using a chemical peel. With this technique, your eye doctor will use an acid called trichloroacetic acid on your skin to cause it to shed its outermost layers. By doing this, you'll be removing the sun-damaged, less vibrant top layers of skin to reveal the newer skin layers beneath. The newer skin cells underneath tend to be more uniformly pigmented and tighter, so you can see an improvement in the appearance of blotchy, loose, or finely wrinkled skin that makes us look older. A chemical peel can also promote the growth of collagen, a support protein for the skin, which can help skin to look less thin.

Chemical peels can be used around the eyes as well as on other parts of the face and body. Sometimes a series of peels is used for best effect. You can discuss with your doctor whether a chemical peel, laser skin resurfacing, or some other rejuvenation technique will work best to address your problem areas.

To have a chemical peel performed, you'll go to your doctor's office where the trichloroacetic acid is applied to your skin for several minutes. You may experience some mild burning or stinging while the acid is applied. Then the chemical is rinsed away and cool compresses and ointment may be applied to your skin. Your skin will look red and raw for five to seven days while your skin is healing. You may wish to avoid high-profile appearances during this healing period.

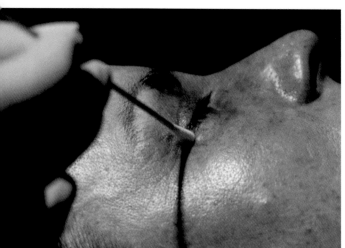

Trichloroacetic acid being applied to the eyelids as a chemical peel.

The most common possible side effect of a chemical peel is that your skin could have brown discoloration afterward. This discoloration is usually, but not always, reversible. The main cause of this side effect is failure to avoid sun exposure after the chemical peel. For this reason, after a chemical peel you must avoid direct sun for six to eight weeks and use a strong, full-spectrum sunscreen when going outside.

Facelifts

While facelifts don't directly treat the aging changes that affect our eyes and eyelids, cosmetic eyelid treatments are sometimes combined with facelifts for people who want a more complete way to look younger. Some eye doctors who specialize in cosmetic eyelid surgery are also trained to perform facelifts. As time passes, gravity causes our facial skin and underlying tissues to droop. Sagging tissues and loose skin can make us look older, so a variety of facelifts are available to surgically enhance our appearance. Two main types of facelifts are the midface lift and lower face lift.

Midface lift

The midface is the area between the lower eyelids and the nasolabial folds, which are the lines from the nose to the corners of the mouth. As we age, this area, like others on our body, can sag and droop. Surgery to lift this area can result in a more youthful facial contour. Sometimes fat is also injected under the facial skin, in combination with a midface lift, to help give a youthful fullness to the features.

Facelifts are more invasive than other cosmetic eyelid procedures, in part because they often require more anesthesia during the procedure. Be sure to feel comfortable with your surgeon and have realistic expectations for your results after you heal. Risks of facelifts, like other surgeries, include bleeding, infection, scarring, and needing further surgery in the future. The eyelids are not typically included in a midface lift, so to surgically enhance this area, a blepharoplasty or brow lift may be needed.

Lower face lift

Gravity can take its toll on the lower face and neck, where loose, sagging tissues can betray our age and the passage of time. The skin of the lower face and neck tends to become looser over time, the fat that provides youthful, natural contours under the skin can shrink, and tissues of the neck can droop with age. With a lower face lift, the neck is often also lifted. In this surgery, the neck muscles are shortened and tightened and excess deposits of fat may be removed.

With extensive cosmetic surgery such as this, it's extremely important to find a surgeon who specializes in facial surgery. Having a doctor who listens to your concerns and expectations, and who takes the time to discuss the tiny details that can affect your appearance, is the most crucial element of successful cosmetic surgery. Similar to a midface lift, risks of surgery may include bleeding, infection, scarring, and needing further surgery in the future. Since the eyelids are not part of a lower face lift, a blepharoplasty or brow lift may also be desired to make the eyes themselves appear more youthful.

Removing eyelid lumps and bumps

As we get older, many of us will have tiny growths on our eyelids or around our eye area. These growths can have a variety of causes, and many are benign and may not bother us at all. Others can be cancerous, however, and should be removed.

MAKING YOUR COSMETIC EYE SURGERY PROCEDURE A SUCCESS

- Find an eye doctor who has experience with the kind of procedure you're considering and with whom you feel at ease.

- During your preoperative visit, ask as many questions as you need to feel comfortable about your procedure.

- Tell your eye doctor about any medical problems you may have (especially infection or bleeding problems) prior to the procedure.

- If you take blood thinners such as aspirin, warfarin, clopidogrel, NSAIDs, vitamin E, or herbs, talk with your eye doctor and family doctor about whether you need to stop these prior to the procedure.

- Tell your eye doctor if you have dry eye problems prior to deciding whether to have the procedure performed.

- Have reasonable expectations for your results; take time to discuss these with your doctor before deciding whether the procedure is right for you.

- Realize that touch-ups or repeat procedures may be necessary.

- Ask ahead of time if you'll need to arrange for someone else to drive you to and from the procedure, particularly if you will be given anesthesia.

- Don't plan high-profile public appearances for yourself while you're in the healing period since it may take time, depending on your type of procedure, for you to recover and look your best.

- Follow your doctor's follow-up instructions religiously. They're designed to optimize your results and protect your new, younger-looking appearance.

- Avoid smoking before the procedure and during the healing period since smoking delays wound healing.

Skin cancer

Skin cancers that affect the eyelids are usually either basal cell carcinomas or squamous cell carcinomas (these terms come from the type of skin cell from which the cancer arises). Rarer and more dangerous skin cancers that can occur in the eye area include melanomas, which start in the pigmented cells of the skin, and sebaceous cell carcinomas, which arise from the oil glands of the eyelid skin. All these skin cancers should be removed if detected, since basal and squamous cell carcinomas may spread to surrounding tissues, and melanomas and sebaceous cell carcinomas can spread to other parts of the body.

Sun exposure is a major risk factor for the development of most eyelid skin cancers. People with fair skin are more prone to developing these skin cancers for this reason. Protecting your eyes from the sun by avoiding sun exposure and wearing sunglasses with ultraviolet protection can reduce your lifetime risk of eyelid skin cancers.

If you notice a bump in your eye area, it may very well be benign if it has been there for a long time without changing. In this case, you don't necessarily need to do anything if it doesn't bother you. If the bump does irritate you because of its location or cosmetic appearance, ask your eye doctor what treatment options are available. However, if your bump has signs that are suggestive of skin cancer, see your eye doctor promptly as a biopsy should be performed to look for signs of cancer.

If your eye doctor thinks that your eye area bump is a skin cancer, removing it entirely is generally the best treatment. Certain eye doctors, called oculoplastic surgeons, specialize in eyelid surgery and this type of treatment. For some eyelid skin cancer patients, their eye doctor may recommend Mohs surgery, or frozen sections to remove the cancer. In these techniques, layers of the cancer are removed one by one and each layer is examined with a microscope during the surgery, thus ensuring that all the cancer cells are removed. Afterward, an oculoplastic surgeon can surgically repair the skin defect that is left after the cancer has been totally removed. For certain eye area cancers that cannot be treated by complete removal, radiation therapy may be useful.

Detecting skin cancer early is key to ensuring that it can be completely removed, thus reducing the risk of recurrence or spread to other areas. Once a cancer has been removed,

---

SIGNS OF SKIN CANCER CAN INCLUDE:

- A new bump on the skin
- A non-healing sore
- A spot that bleeds or crusts repeatedly
- A growth that distorts the eyelid structure or causes eyelashes to be missing
- A mole that is tender or bleeds
- A mole that looks irregular or changes its size, shape, or color
- A persistently inflamed, thickened eyelid edge

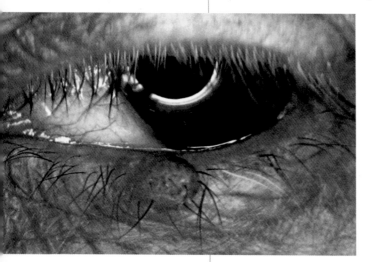

Basal cell carcinoma on the lower eyelid. The nodule, or bump, disrupts the normal eyelash line, which is suggestive of skin cancer in this location.

it's necessary to follow up regularly with your eye doctor to make sure it doesn't recur, and to look for other skin cancers that could develop in the future.

Ocular prostheses (artificial eyes)

While we all hope to have two healthy eyes that allow us to see well and look normal throughout our lives, not everyone is fortunate enough to achieve this goal. Most people even with a blind eye can keep their natural eyeball, but in some cases, an eye may need to be removed. This can happen after a severe injury, to treat some eye cancers, to alleviate pain in a blind eye, to treat a severe infection in the eye, or for cosmetic improvement of a blind and disfigured eye.

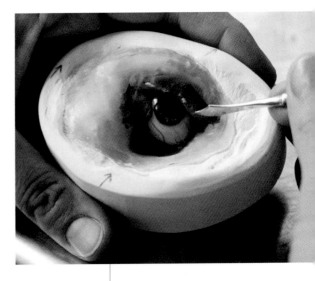

An ocularist at work crafting a realistic-looking ocular prosthesis.

If an eyeball is removed with surgery, the eye surgeon typically places a ball-like implant in the eye socket to take the place of the eyeball. This spherical implant can be made of silicone, hydroxyapatite, polyethylene, or alumina, and is covered with the patient's own tissues. In many cases, the muscles that were attached to the natural eyeball are reattached to the implant so it can move like a natural eyeball. After several weeks, while the implant heals, an eye care professional (an ocularist) makes a prosthesis, or artificial eye. She will paint the prosthesis to match the other eye, and its shape will be custom molded to fit behind the eyelid and in front of the implant. Sometimes a peg is placed to connect the implant to the prosthesis so the artificial eye will appear to move more naturally, since the eye muscles move the implant. Prostheses can be easily removed for cleaning, and most people sleep with them in place. Prostheses can last for decades.

Ocularists are artists who make artificial eyes look like real eyes. These artificial eyes, however, provide no vision and serve only a cosmetic and structural purpose.

Without a natural eyeball, the eye socket and eyelids can change their shape over time, so the fit of the prosthesis can change. If you have a prosthesis, it's important to follow up regularly with your eye surgeon and ocularist to make sure the prosthesis fits well, and the implant and its overlying tissues stay in place. Many of us may not be used to the idea of an artificial eye, and losing an eye can have a deep psychological impact. However, eyeballs that have to be removed usually have very serious problems, making the surgery necessary. Especially in the case of blind painful eyes, many people are significantly happier after the eye is removed because this relieves their pain. It may be difficult for some to become accustomed to the concept of an artificial eye, but most people adjust well to this with time.

8

For Further Vision

Here are some useful pieces of information that can help you as you peruse this book. You'll find a section on common eye myths, a section on how to put in eyedrops properly, and a list of commonly prescribed eyedrops, explaining how to use them and their side effects. Also included is a list of suggested questions for you to use as a guide in preparing for eye surgery.

Common eye myths dispelled

All of us have heard old wives' tales about our eyes, but it can be difficult at times to separate fact from fiction. Here are some common myths that we all may have encountered and the reasons why they shouldn't be believed.

Do eye exercises improve your vision?

You may see commercials for eye exercises or computer programs that are designed to improve your vision and reduce your need for glasses. In reality, your refractive error, or need for glasses, is mostly set by your genes, and is determined by the shape of your eyeball. So exercises will not change your refractive error and will not make your vision better. The only exercise that can help some people who suffer from convergence insufficiency, or difficulty aligning and focusing both eyes together to look at near objects, is pencil push-ups (see chapter 3).

Does too much reading or watching television permanently damage your eyes?

Think of your eye as a digital camera and your brain as a computer. Your eye captures images that you see, like a digital camera, and sends that visual information to your brain, which functions as the computer to which the camera's images are uploaded. Your brain then processes those images so you can actually "see" them.

Just as a camera is not damaged by what it takes a picture of, your eye is not damaged by what you look at. Though it's possible to experience uncomfortable eyestrain, which is often due to eye dryness, by staring at a book or television, this does not permanently damage your eyes.

Something to note is that the refractive error of children's eyes, which are still growing and developing, may be partly influenced by how they

TEST YOUR
Eye Q:

True or False?

Children who play outdoors may have lower rates of nearsightedness than those who mostly stay indoors.

True

A study conducted by researcher, Dr. Kathryn Rose at the University of Sydney in 2008, found that outdoor activity reduces the prevalence of myopia in children.

READING

Although the eyestrain that you can feel after reading, watching television, or using the computer is generally not dangerous for your eyes, it can be bothersome. If your eyes feel irritated or itchy, or if you notice slightly blurrier vision in both eyes after you've been staring at a book or a monitor for a while, try these tips.

- **Close your eyes to let your own tears moisten the surface of your eyes.**
- **Put an artificial teardrop in each eye to moisten them.**
- **Look at a distant scene or object for a couple of minutes to relax the muscle inside your eye that helps you focus up close.**
- **Get up, stretch, and do something else for a little while before you try reading or looking at the television or monitor again.**
- **The next time you sit down to read, watch television, or use the computer, put an artificial teardrop in each eye before you start.**

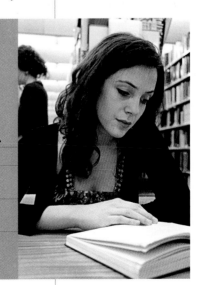

are used. It's thought that although genetics largely determines a person's refractive error, some studies have shown that spending significant time reading and doing close-up work may make children more prone to developing nearsightedness.

Does wearing glasses make your eyes weaker?

Just as reading or watching television does not damage your eyes, wearing glasses with your correct prescription doesn't harm them either. In fact, the most important measure of your level of vision assumes that your vision is "best corrected," meaning that you can use whatever glasses you need to help you see your best. Wearing the appropriate glasses prescription does not make your eyes lazy; in fact, your vision will be better if you are wearing the glasses that you need. Even wearing a glasses prescription that is not quite perfect won't permanently damage your eyes, although in some instances it can cause eyestrain or headache.

> If your eyesight is defective then you need to wear glasses to correct your sight and improve vision.

However, for children who need glasses to correct their refractive error, wearing the correct glasses prescription is crucial. Blurry vision in a child, whether it's caused by not wearing the necessary glasses or wearing an incorrect prescription, can cause problems because the child's brain is still developing its neural connections to the eyes. In the worst case, if the eyes can only send blurry images to the brain, then the brain may not develop those connections properly. This can result in amblyopia, or lazy eye, which can cause permanent decreased vision in the future if it is not adequately treated in childhood.

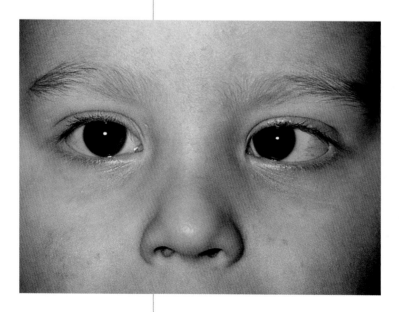

A three-year-old boy with a squint in his left eye. If a strabismus is left untreated it can have damaging consequences to the child's eyesight.

Do children just outgrow strabismus (crossed eyes)?

Some people think that if a young child has eyes that cross in or turn out, this will correct itself as the child gets older. It is true that newborns may have unsteady eye alignment as their vision develops, but after about four months of age, any strabismus is concerning and should be evaluated by an eye doctor. Children do not outgrow strabismus, and having eye misalignment in childhood is a risk factor for developing amblyopia, or lazy eye (see chapter 3). Strabismus can also be a symptom of more serious eye problems, so it's crucial to have an eye doctor perform a thorough eye exam to look for any other abnormalities.

Does eating carrots improve your vision?

Carrots are a good source of beta-carotene, which is converted by the body into vitamin A. Vitamin A plays an important role in how the cells that make up the retina function. In cases of vitamin A deficiency, night blindness is a common first sign, and more severe blindness can result later on. In the developing world, vitamin A deficiency is not uncommon. In developed countries, however, vitamin A deficiency is quite rare in healthy individuals. Eating carrots, or other foods that contain large amounts of beta carotene, will not make your vision any better, unless you are already deficient in vitamin A. Chapter 5 has more information on vitamins and supplements to help improve your vision.

> Eating carrots can only improve a person's eyesight if they are already deficient in vitamin A.

The Age-Related Eye Disease Study results recommend high-dose beta-carotene in combination with other vitamins and minerals to reduce the risk that certain types of dry macular degeneration will progress to the more aggressive wet form of the disease (see chapter 3). Even in this case, though, these vitamins are taken to lessen the chance of vision worsening; they will not improve your vision. Of note, in smokers, high doses of beta-carotene have been linked to an increased risk of lung cancer.

Are tea bags and cucumbers good for eye puffiness?

Many of us have read magazine articles that advise us to put moist tea bags or cucumber slices on our eyelids to reduce puffiness. The problem with doing so is that food may contain bacteria, which we don't want to get in our eyes. While bacteria are everywhere in our environment, putting a possible bacterial source directly against our eyes is not recommended. This is especially true for people who wear contact lenses, which make their eyes slightly more susceptible to bacterial infections.

OPTICAL ILLUSION

Cucumbers are over 90 percent water and the rest is mostly inert fiber. However, cucumber slices do sometimes reduce puffiness. That's because they are cold! It is the cold (not the cucumber) that shrinks the swelling by constricting blood vessels and thus reducing inflow of fluid into soft tissues. You can get the same results with a washcloth dipped in cold water.

Some fashion magazines have also recommended using hemorrhoid creams on the eyelids to reduce puffiness. This is because these creams contain medicines that constrict the blood vessels (hemorrhoids are enlarged blood vessels). By constricting the blood vessels in the eyelids, this may help reduce swelling. However, any effect these creams have on eyelid puffiness and swelling is minimal and temporary. These creams are not formulated for the sensitive eye area, so they can irritate the eyes and the thin skin of the eyelids. Also, some hemorrhoid creams contain steroid medicines, which can cause or worsen cataracts and glaucoma if used near the eyes.

If you want to soothe your eyes and potentially help their puffiness temporarily, try using cool compresses. To make a compress, wring a clean washcloth out under cool running water, close your eyes, and put the washcloth on your eyelids for a few minutes.

OPTICAL ILLUSION

Laser treatments performed to control diabetic retinopathy or to lower eye pressure in glaucoma will not actually improve your vision. The goal of these laser treatments is to preserve the vision you currently have as much as possible.

The goal of lasers to treat an after-cataract film is to improve your vision; it is not designed to reduce your need for glasses.

Are all eye lasers designed to improve your vision and reduce your need for glasses?

When many of us hear "eye laser," we immediately think of refractive surgery, where lasers are used to reduce one's need for glasses or contact lenses. However, there are a number of other types of laser treatments that are used to treat eye problems and diseases and do not affect a person's refractive error, or need for glasses. Examples of these treatments include: laser to the retina to control certain types of diabetic retinopathy, laser to the iris to treat or prevent angle-closure glaucoma, laser to the eye's internal drainage area to lower eye pressure in open-angle glaucoma, and laser to treat an "after-cataract," or film that can form behind an artificial lens implant after cataract surgery. These lasers can have a varying effect on your vision, and they are not likely to change your glasses prescription. See chapter 2 for futher information on laser surgery.

Is all cataract surgery performed with a laser?

Cataract surgery techniques have changed and improved immensely over

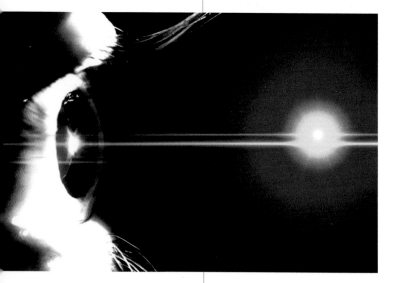

the last 25 years, and most cataract surgery in the developed world today is performed with specialized ultrasound machines, not with lasers. The ultrasound machine breaks up the cloudy cataract lens and removes it in small pieces rather than removing the whole cataract intact, which means that modern cataract surgery requires a much smaller incision and therefore less healing time than older surgical techniques.

A laser is used, however, to remove the "after-cataract" film that can form behind the artificial lens implant at any point after cataract surgery (see chapter 3).

Do macular degeneration and glaucoma lead to total blindness?

The good news about these two diseases is that they do not often lead to total blindness in both eyes. In the case of macular degeneration, this disease by itself never leads to total blindness. This is because macular degeneration only affects the macula, which is the center of the retina responsible for your central vision. Therefore, the peripheral retina, which is responsible for your side vision, is not affected. Even people who suffer from advanced macular degeneration generally have enough side vision to walk around without assistance.

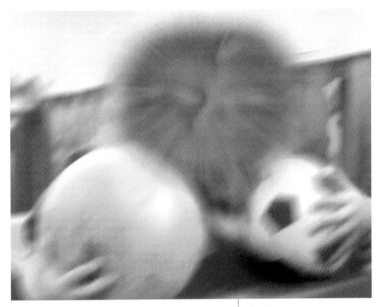

While macular degeneration can affect your central vision, your side vision is generally well preserved.

In the case of glaucoma, most people do not go blind in both eyes. This varies, depending on the type of glaucoma. Open-angle glaucoma, which is the most common type, tends to be a slow disease that only leads to blindness in very aggressive cases. If it is diagnosed reasonably early in its course and well-treated, total blindness in both eyes is quite rare. With acute angle-closure glaucoma, the risk of blindness is somewhat higher because eye pressure can rise quite high very quickly, and this can permanently damage the vision within hours or days if untreated. However, acute angle-closure attacks hardly ever happen in both eyes at the same time, and if treated promptly and properly, the risk of total blindness in both eyes is fortunately low. Both these diseases are discussed in more depth in chapter 3.

Are eyedrops that make the whites of your eyes whiter good to use?

In general, it is not recommended to use over-the-counter eyedrops that are designed to whiten your eyes or remove redness. These medicated eyedrops, which differ from artificial teardrops, contain chemicals that constrict the blood vessels in the conjunctiva, or tissue that overlies the white part of your eyeball. When the blood vessels constrict, they appear smaller, thus reducing the appearance of redness. This change is temporary, and when the medication wears off, the blood vessels can rebound and enlarge,

For those who use artificial tears more than four times per day, consider using preservative-free varieties. These tend to be less irritating with frequent usage.

making the eyes look even redder than before. Also, eye redness can be a sign of a more serious eye problem, and temporarily hiding the redness with this type of eyedrop can mask the need to see an eye doctor.

If you want to use eyedrops to moisturize your eyes and help them to feel more comfortable, try over-the-counter artificial teardrops first. Artificial teardrops do not contain the medicine that constricts blood vessels. You can use artificial teardrops as often as you like, particularly if they are preservative-free.

Lubricating gels or ointments used at bedtime can be particularly useful to keep your eyes moistened overnight, making them more comfortable in the morning.

It is useful to store your eyedrops in the refrigerator to keep them fresh. Since refrigerated eyedrops are cold, it's easier to tell whether they enter your eye as compared with non-refrigerated eyedrops.

When putting in eyedrops, is it possible to get too many eyedrops in at one time?

The eyeball and its surrounding eyelids can only hold about the volume of a single drop of liquid. Therefore, if you put in more than one eyedrop in your eye at a time, the excess liquid will simply run down your cheek. So if you are not sure if an eyedrop actually went into your eye, put in another right away because it's not possible to overdose. It's better to have the excess drop run down your face than not to get enough of a medicated eyedrop.

OPTICAL ILLUSION

While your eye doctor can recommend whether or not you should have eye surgery, the decision is actually up to you. Although many people are comfortable doing what their doctor tells them to do, you must understand the pros and cons of the surgery in order for you to assess whether you need it and to feel comfortable about your decision.

Questions to ask your doctor in preparation for eye surgery

While the thought of eye surgery can be scary, many millions of people worldwide have undergone successful eye surgery. Finding out as much as you can in advance about your or a loved one's eye surgery is helpful in preparing for it. Feel free to ask your eye surgeon as many questions as necessary for you to feel comfortable about your operation. The following list contains some sample questions with explanations that may be useful to you and your eye doctor, as you consider your decision. For further information on eye surgery refer back to chapter 2 (refractive surgery), chapter 3 (cataract surgery) and chapter 7 (cosmetic surgery).

How many of these procedures have you done?

While the absolute number of surgeries your eye surgeon has performed may not directly influence your surgery, it may be useful for you to know not only how experienced your surgeon is, but also how common your type of surgery is. While operations such as cataract surgery are fairly commonplace, other types of surgery are performed less often. With common surgeries, your postoperative course may be easy to predict, whereas with rarer surgeries your postoperative recovery may be somewhat more difficult to foresee.

What are my risks and benefits for this surgery?

When you decide on eye surgery, it should be a joint decision between you and your eye doctor. She may recommend the appropriate course of action, but ultimately you'll have to make the final decision about whether surgery is right for you. Usually, you'll arrive at this decision by weighing the potential risks and benefits. Your eye doctor will help you identify the risks and benefits that apply to your situation so you can carefully weigh the pros and cons of surgery.

> If you have doubts or concerns about a recommended surgery or treatment, it never hurts to get a second opinion, as long as your situation is not urgent.

What is the expected success rate?

For the most common types of eye surgery, there are estimates of what percentage of people do well with the surgery and what typical complication rates may be. Your eye doctor will be able to tailor these statistics to your situation, since not everyone has the same characteristics as patients enrolled in medical studies. Ask your doctor whether his rates of success are similar to those in the scientific literature. Also keep in mind that complications vary widely. Some are mild and don't end up having a lasting effect on your vision, while other more serious complications have the potential to affect your vision long-term. Fortunately the likelihood of these serious complications tends to be lower than the likelihood of milder complications, which may get better with treatment and with time.

What type of anesthesia is best for my surgery?

In some cases, you and your eye doctor may have a choice about the anesthesia you are given. In general, it's better for your overall health to have less anesthesia rather than more. For instance, if a procedure can be performed under local anesthesia, it's usually healthier to go this route rather than having general anesthesia where you are put completely to sleep. Certain factors influence how much anesthesia you'll need for a surgery, such as potential pain during the procedure, how still you need to stay during surgery, the length of surgery, and your other medical problems. Your eye doctor will help you assess your particular situation in order to decide which type of anesthesia you will most easily tolerate while also providing the safest setting for him to perform your operation.

What are my other options?

Even if you and your eye doctor decide together to proceed with your planned surgery, it's good to know what the alternatives are. If there are other non-surgical options that you haven't tried, your eye doctor may give you reasons why surgery would be a better choice. In some situations, there is more than one right answer about which type of surgery to perform, so you should be informed about why your eye doctor has chosen your particular surgery to be your best option. Finally, for some people, surgery isn't an attractive idea, so choosing a less aggressive treatment may be preferable, as long as they understand the risks and benefits of doing so.

Are there any experimental therapies for my condition that are currently being tested?

Fortunately scientists are constantly making progress and discovering new breakthroughs in medicine. In eye care, there are always new procedures, devices, and medicines being tested and studied at various stages. These newer technologies tend to become widely used once they are approved and then used regularly to make sure that they stand the test of time. For instance, multifocal intraocular lens implants used in cataract surgery are currently being improved and newer versions tend to work even better than older versions. Some surgeons choose to offer these newer lens implants, while others prefer to wait for even better lens implants to be developed before using them. In many cases, it's not right or wrong to opt for a newer technology over an older, more established one, but you should be informed about the available options so you can make the best choice for yourself with your eye doctor's help.

Most eye surgeries are performed while you lie flat on your back.

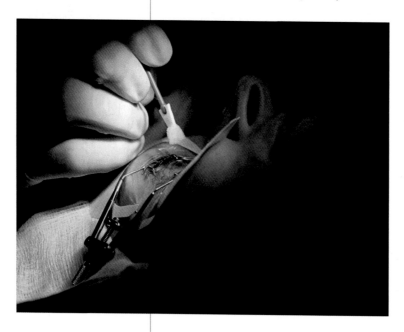

If I can't lie flat on my back when I sleep at night, will this affect my eye surgery?

Many eye surgeries are typically performed with you lying on your back so your eye is facing up to the ceiling. Be sure to let your eye doctor know if you have another medical problem that makes it difficult for you to lie still in this position. In some cases, propping up your neck or knees with extra padding or pillows during surgery can help you to be more comfortable while still allowing your surgeon to work on your eye. Also, your anesthetist may be able to control your other medical problems (by giving pain medicine for back pain, for example) during surgery so that you are able to lie on your back more easily.

Should I stop my blood thinner prior to surgery, and when should I resume it?

If you take aspirin, clopidogrel bisulfate (Plavix), warfarin (Coumadin), or other blood thinners including herbal varieties, be sure to ask your eye doctor if you should discontinue this medication prior to your eye surgery. Once again, your doctor will weigh the risks to the rest of your body of stopping your blood thinner versus the risk of your eye having a serious bleeding problem during or after surgery if you keep taking the medication. If you take the blood thinner because you've had a stroke, blood clot, or heart attack, for instance, your eye doctor may ask your primary care provider or internist to help make this decision because these are serious health problems that could recur. If the risk of bleeding with the eye surgery is low, then your eye doctor may decide that you are better off continuing to take the medication. However, if the risk of bleeding is significant, then your eye doctor may ask you to stop the blood thinner prior to surgery. Typically, aspirin is stopped 10–14 days prior to surgery, since it takes that amount of time to clear out of your system, while clopidogrel bisulfate and warfarin are stopped 3–5 days prior to surgery. Don't forget to find out when you should resume these medications, which may be as soon as the day after surgery in some cases.

Some people have to take warfarin for serious medical conditions that put them at risk for major health problems if they stop this blood thinner. If you are in this category and yet you need to undergo eye surgery that has a substantial risk of bleeding, there is a potential compromise that can be helpful. In conjunction with your primary care provider, your eye doctor may ask you to stop your warfarin several days prior to surgery but then replace it with enoxaparin sodium (Lovenox), which is a blood-thinning medication that is injected under your skin twice daily. Enoxaparin sodium will keep your blood thin while the warfarin is clearing out of your system. Because this is a complicated regimen, be sure that your eye doctor and

OPTICAL ILLUSION

In diabetics with diabetic retinopathy, it seems logical that taking aspirin (a blood thinner) would increase the risk of bleeding in the eye. However, a large research study did not find any effect of aspirin on disease severity or bleeding risk in people affected by diabetic retinopathy.

If you are taking aspirin or any other blood thinners, consult your doctor before surgery before continuing the medication.

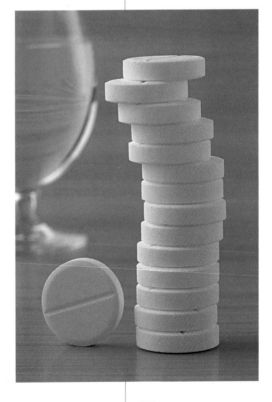

primary care provider are communicating clearly with you and with each other about how you should be taking these blood thinning medications.

Will my medical insurance or government health plan cover this surgery?

If you have a typical medical insurance plan, most surgeries that are performed for the health of your eyes (that is, surgeries that are medically necessary) will be covered. Of course, not all insurance and government health plans are the same, so you need to check with your insurer to be certain of this prior to undergoing surgery. Remember that you may have a deductible or co-pay as well.

Refractive surgery and cosmetic eyelid surgery are typically not covered by medical insurance, so you need to be aware that you will probably be required to pay for these types of procedures on your own. Ask your eye doctor's office about the cost of these procedures well in advance of deciding whether or not to have them performed.

What can I do to prepare for my surgery?

Some eye doctors will ask you to start eyedrops prior to surgery, so make sure you have the prescription for these in advance, if applicable. Discuss any blood thinner use with your eye doctor. Depending on the timing of your surgery and the type of anesthesia used, your eye doctor may instruct you not to eat or drink after midnight of the night before surgery. On the day of surgery, make sure to wash your face and avoid wearing eye makeup. Arrange to have someone drive you to and from the surgery that day. Remember to ask any questions about the surgery in advance of the actual surgery, if possible. This way, you will minimize any unexpected surprises.

> In many cases, using your prescribed eyedrops as directed after surgery can make the difference between having a successful outcome and having less-than-perfect results.

How long is my expected recovery?

Your recovery time will vary depending on the type of surgery you have, and while your eye doctor can give you a general time frame, everyone heals differently so your recovery may be somewhat longer or shorter than the next person's. For many types of eye surgery, your vision in the operated eye may be blurry as the eye heals, so remember to ask how quickly it is expected to improve. This is especially important if you have good vision in only one eye and are planning to undergo surgery in that eye; if your vision is blurry while your good eye heals, you may need to arrange help at home or more time off from work during that period. Also, after some eye surgeries, your glasses prescription may change. In this case, your vision may seem blurry in the operated eye until things have stabilized enough for your eye doctor to give you a new glasses prescription.

What will my activity restrictions be during recovery time?

In order to reduce your risk of complications from some types of eye surgery, your eye doctor may ask you to avoid strenuous activity while you are healing. Ask your doctor when you can resume your regular exercise program. You should also find out whether you need to avoid getting water in your eyes or for how long you should avoid swimming, if that is an activity you pursue. Your eye doctor can tell you if you need to keep your eye covered with glasses, sunglasses, or a plastic shield while you heal. If you wear contact lenses, ask your doctor when it is safe to resume wearing them. If you plan to travel during the healing period, ask your eye doctor if this is acceptable. Your eye doctor may prefer that you stay local after surgery in case of any urgent complications that may occur. Also, for some types of retinal surgery, in particular, flying is not allowed while the eye is healing. Some retinal surgeries require you to maintain a certain head position for much of the healing period in order for the surgery to be successful, so you need to know in advance how this will affect your daily routine.

OPTICAL ILLUSION

The Internet is a great source of information about medical conditions, but keep in mind that not all the facts come from reliable sources. Some Web sites that seem informative are in fact set up by companies who are trying to sell a particular product. So if you are researching your eye surgery on the Internet, verify your findings with your eye doctor.

It's important to know how you can help your eye heal during your recovery period, so besides knowing what to avoid, be sure to receive clear instructions from your surgeon about what you should do to help after surgery. Most important, use your postoperative eyedrops faithfully, since these can be crucial for proper healing, and keep your scheduled follow-up visits.

What particular problems should I look out for while I heal from surgery?

In general, if you notice anything out of the ordinary while you are recovering from eye surgery, it is best to have it checked earlier rather than later. Many complications are much more easily dealt with if they are diagnosed before they become more serious later on. It's also better to be safe than sorry, so even if you're not sure if a symptom that you notice is a problem, it's best to call your eye doctor to ask. Examples of typical problems that require urgent medical attention are serious eye pain and worsening vision, although there may be other problems that your eye doctor may warn you about that are specific to your type of surgery. Make sure you know how to contact your eye doctor or the covering doctor, particularly if a problem arises at night or on the weekend.

Where can I find out more information about my surgery?

Many eye doctors have literature or hand-outs that they can give you so you can read about your surgery in advance. Your eye doctor may also recommend Web sites containing useful information about your particular eye problem so that you can do research on your own and maximize your understanding about your eye health.

Ocular medications

Eye medications are used to diagnose, treat and prevent eye diseases. There are a bewildering number of eye medications available on prescription and over-the-counter. Artificial tears and ocular decongestants are most commonly available as over-the-counter eye drops. Eye drops and ointments are the most usual ways to medicate the eye. Other types of administration are oral (tablets, capsules, liquids), intravenous and local injections.

Eyedrops

When an eye care professional recommends the use of eyedrops, sometimes patients express concern about how to properly instill the medications. In this section, we will go over a step-by-step technique that patients can follow when administering their eyedrops to assure that the drops properly get into the eye.

Administering eyedrops

While administering eyedrops may seem like an easy task, many patients actually struggle quite a bit with getting eyedrops into their eyes. If your eye care professional has recommended that you use eyedrops for glaucoma, to treat inflammation in your eye, or for other purposes, it is very important that the prescribed eyedrops get into your eye. Below is a step-by-step technique that can be useful in helping you with eyedrop administration.

- Begin by washing your hands with soap and water.
- Gently shake the bottle of eyedrops you are planning to use.
- Unscrew the cap of the eyedrop bottle.
- Tilt your head back and gaze upward or recline in a chair so your looking up at the ceiling.
- With your dominant hand, grasp the bottle of eyedrops with your thumb and forefinger and bring the bottle toward your eye.

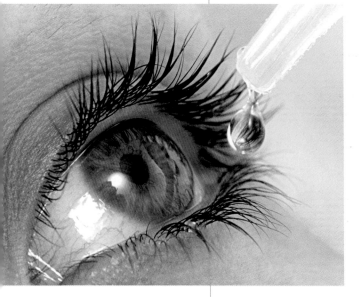

The correct technique for administering eyedrops.

- With the little finger of your dominant hand, pull down the lower eyelid of the eye you are about to place the eyedrop into.
- With the bottle held above your open eye, squeeze the bottle so that one drop goes out of the bottle onto the surface of your eye.
- Be sure not to let the tip of the eyedrop container touch the surface of your eye when administering the eyedrops.
- Once the eyedrop has been placed in your eye, let go of your lower eyelid and close your eyes.
- With your eye closed, take the index finger of your dominant hand and place it on the lacrimal sac, which is the small bump located in the corner of your eye between the eye and nose. Hold your finger there for 2 minutes. This reduces the amount of eyedrop going into your nose and down your throat.

If you try putting an eyedrop into your eye and are unsuccessful, place a second drop into your eye. If you continue to struggle with placing an eyedrop into your eye, be sure to inform your eye care professional, and she can work with you to make sure you are administering the drops properly.

Alternatively, some patients seek assistance from a friend or family member with administering eyedrops.

Daily eyedrop reminder chart

If you have been prescribed multiple kinds of eyedrops either for use after eye surgery or for other chronic eye problems such as glaucoma, it may be confusing to remember how and when to use them. A handy chart is included on the next page to help you keep your eyedrops organized.

To use the chart:

1 Photocopy the chart so you'll have a blank copy to write on.
2 Fill it in using thick, dark marker so that it's easy to read, particularly if your vision is not perfect.
3 In the first row of the first column labeled "eyedrop," write the name of the medication.
4 In the second column labeled "cap color," write the color of the cap because it is often easier to identify this than to read the eyedrop name on the bottle label.
5 In the third column labeled "which eye (R/L/both)," write a large "R" for right eye or an "L" for left eye.

In the columns labeled "breakfast," "lunch," "dinner," and "bedtime," place check marks to indicate when the drops should be used. For example, a drop that is used twice daily might have check marks placed in the breakfast and dinner columns.

DAILY EYEDROP REMINDER CHART

Brand name	Cap color	Which eye (R/L/both)	Breakfast	Lunch	Dinner	Bedtime

Commonly Prescribed Eyedrops

The next few pages list frequently prescribed eyedrops for various ocular conditions along with information about why these medications are prescribed and some of the common side effects that are known to be associated with these various eyedrops. While these lists cover many of the generic and brand name ocular medications, the list of medications and side effects are by no means comprehensive. Whenever your eye care provider prescribes a new eyedrop for you to use, you should speak with her about the benefits and possible side effects associated with the particular medication before taking it. Please refer back to chapter 5 for further information on eye problems such as itchy eyes, dry eyes, and inflamed eyes.

CORTICOSTEROID EYEDROPS			
OCULAR INFLAMMATION		INTRAOCULAR INFLAMMATION	
Generic name*	Brand name	Generic name*	Brand name
Diclofenac	Voltaren	Prednisolone acetate	Pred Forte, Econo Pred
Flurbiprofen	Ocufen	Prednisolone phosphate	AK- Pred, Imflamase
Ketorolac	Acular	Dexamethasone phosphate	Tobradex, Maxidex
Nepatenac	Nevanac	Fluoromethalone	FML
Suprofen	Profenal	Loteprednol	Alrex, Lotemax
		Rimexolone	Vexol

*May be sold under a different name, depending on the country where you live.

Notes
These eyedrops are used to decrease or prevent swelling and inflammation after cataract surgery or other intraocular surgical procedures.

They may also be used for eye allergies.

Notes
Corticosteroid eyedrops are frequently administered after eye surgery to help reduce inflammation.

These medications often need to be gradually reduced to prevent the inflammation from returning.

If you require chronic use of corticosteroids, your eye care professional needs to monitor you carefully for the development of cataracts or glaucoma.

EYEDROPS FOR GLAUCOMA

Generic name*	Brand name	Bottle cap color	How often to take**	Side effects	Comments
Timolol Betaxolol Levobunolol Carteolol	Timoptic Betoptic Betagan Ocupress	Yellow	Once or twice a day	Difficulty with breathing, slow heart rate, low blood pressure, lethargy, depression	If you have asthma or chronic obstructive pulmonary disease, these products should be used with caution.
Pilocarpine	Pilopine HS, Isopto Carpine, Pilocar, Pilogel	Green	Four times a day	Brow ache, blurry vision, small pupils, redness of the conjunctiva	Comes in different strengths from 0.5% to 6%
Dorzolamide Brinzolamide Acetazolamide Methazolamide	Trusopt Azopt Diamox Neptazane	Orange	Twice a day	Numbness and tingling, altered taste, kidney stones, loss of appetite	Diamox and Neptazane have more side effects than Azopt or Trusopt.
Dorzolamide and Timolol	Cosopt	White	Twice a day	Blurry vision, difficulty with breathing, slow heart rate	Cosopt may be harmful to an unborn baby.
Brimonidine	Alphagan-P	Purple	Twice a day	Redness of the conjunctiva	Should not be used for young children.
Latanoprost Bimatoprost Travaprost	Xalatan Lumigan Travatan	Green	Once at bedtime	Eyelash growth, changes in iris color, redness of the conjunctiva	

*May be sold under a different name, depending on the country where you live.

** This is the frequency these medications are usually administered. Check with your eye care professional before use.

Notes
These are common glaucoma medications in the United States. In other countries other agents may be available, (for example, Xalacom).

COMMON EYEDROPS TO TREAT EYE INFECTIONS

Antibiotic type	Brand name	Use	Comments
Aminoglycosides	Neomycin, Gentamicin, Tobramycin	Bacterial conjunctivitis, keratitis (infection of the cornea), dacrocystitis (infection of the tear drainage system), blepharitis	Redness and irritation of the skin around the eyes
Antivirals	Trifluorothymidine (Viroptic), Vidarabine (Vira-A), Acyclovir	Treats corneal infections caused by the Herpes virus	
Erythromycin	Romycin Ilotycin Many others	Bacterial conjunctivitis and blepharitis	Relatively inexpensive, ointment can temporarily cause blurring to the vision
Fluoroquinolones	Ofloxacin, (Ocuflox) Vigamox, Zyma	Broad spectrum (kills most types of bacteria) antibiotics that are frequently prescribed after eye surgery to prevent infection	Can be expensive
Trimethoprim-polymyxin B	Polytrim	Bacterial conjunctivitis, blepharitis	

Other medications for your eyes

There are a range of eye drops and oral medications used to treat itchy eyes if you are suffering from an allergy. The chart on the following page list some of the most common drugs available. However, remember that it is important to consult your eye doctor or an eye care professional before beginning a course of any new medicines.

During an eye examination, an eye care professional will administer certain medications for a variety of reasons such as measuring eye pressure, dilating pupils or assessing the blood supply to the eye. The chart on page 169 will help you prepare for this.

ALLERGY MEDICATIONS

EYEDROPS		ORAL MEDICATIONS	
Generic name*	Brand name	Generic name*	Brand name
Cromolyn	Crolom	Azelastine	Astelin
Emedastine	Emadine	Brompheniramine	Bromphen, Dimetane, Dimetapp, Nasahist, Robitussin
Ketotifen fumarate	Zaditor	Carbinozamine	Palgic
Levocabastine	Livostin	Certirizine	Zyrtec, Zyrtec D
Lodoxamide	Alomide	Chlorpheniramine	Singlet
Naphazoline	Naphcon	Clemastine	Allerhist, Tavist
Nedocromil	Alocril	Desloratadine	Clarinex, Clarinex D
Olopatadine	Patanol	Dimenhydrinate	Dramamine
Oxymetazoline	Visine	Diphenhydramine	Benadryl, Nytol, Sominex
Pemirolast	Alamast	Doxylamine	Vicks NyQuil, Alka-Seltzer Plus Night-Time Cold Medicine
Pheniramine / antazoline	Avil Vasocon-A	Fexofenadine	Allergra, Allerga D
		Levocetirizine	Xyzal
		Loratadine	Alavert, Claritin, Claritin D
		Tecastemizole	Soltara

*May be sold under a different name, depending on the country where you live.

Notes
Frequent or prolonged use of naphazoline (Naphcon)/or oxymetazoline (Visine) can worsen the redness from allergic conjunctivitis.

Notes
This is only a sample of the many oral antihistamines on the market.

These medications may be used to ease itchy eyes caused by seasonal allergies, allergic conjunctivitis, motion sickness, or insomnia.

Side effects include drowsiness, blurred vision, dry mouth, bitter taste, nausea/vomiting, and difficulty urinating.

Speak with your doctor before using these products if you have glaucoma, enlarged prostate, or thyroid disease.

COMMON MEDICATIONS USED DURING EYE EXAMINATIONS

Medication name	Use	Side effects	Comments
Fluorescein strips	Measuring the eye pressure		
Indocyanine green	Injected into the veins to assess the blood supply to the back of the eye	Dizziness, nausea, skin rash	If you are allergic to iodine or shellfish, you can develop a serious allergic reaction to this medication. If you have kidney or liver problems, you may not be able to receive this medication.
Intravenous fluorescein	Injected into the veins to assess the blood vessels in the eye	Nausea and vomiting, dizziness, temporary yellowing of the skin and urine for 24 hours after the test, skin rash, itchy skin	This test is useful in assessing bleeding, swelling, or scar tissue in the retina.
Mydriacyl (tropicamide) Cyclogyl (cyclopentolate)	Dilates the pupil for an eye examination	Blurry vision, glaucoma, fever, increased heart rate, flushing of the skin	Tropicamide is frequently used to dilate the eyes for eye examinations; the dilation usually wears off in 4-6 hours. Cyclopentolate is often used for dilated eye examinations in children.
Phenylephrine	Dilates the pupil for an eye examination	Increased heart rate, increased blood pressure	Often used with tropicamide or cyclopentolate to dilate the eyes for an examination
Proparacaine	Numbs the eye so it can be examined	Chronic use can lead to damage to the surface of the eye	
Tetracaine	Numbs the eye so it can be examined	Chronic use can lead to damage to the surface of the eye	

Additional Resources

USA

About Cataract Surgery
In 2008 the Medical Management Services Group, L.L.C. introduced this Web site to provide patients with access to commercially unbiased information about cataracts, cataract surgery, cataract surgeons, lens implants and cataract surgery centers.
www.aboutcataractsurgery.com

The Eye Digest
Published by the University of Illinois Eye and Ear Infirmary Physicians
www.agingeye.net

The American Foundation for the Blind
The American Foundation for the Blind (AFB) is a national nonprofit that expands possibilities for people with vision loss.
Help Line:
1-800-AFB-LINE (232-5463)
Phone: (212) 502-7600
E-mail: afbinfo@afb.net
www.afb.org

EyeCare America
Founded in 1985, EyeCare America is a public service foundation of the American Academy of Ophthalmology.
Seniors EyeCare Program
1-800-222-EYES (3937)
AMD EyeCare Program
1-800-324-EYES (3937)
Diabetes EyeCare Program
1-800-272-EYES (3937)
Glaucoma EyeCare Program
1-800-391-EYES (3937)
Children's EyeCare Program
1-877-887-6327
www.eyecareamerica.org

Glossary of Eye Terminology
Taken from the Dictionary of Eye Terminology, by Barbara Cassin.
www.eyeglossary.net

Lighthouse International
Founded in 1905, Lighthouse International is the leading non-profit organization worldwide dedicated to preserving vision and to helping people of all ages overcome the challenges of vision loss.
Phone: (212) 821-9200 / (800) 829-0500
Fax: (212) 821-9707
TTY: (212) 821-9713
www.lighthouse.org

The Merck Manuals
Established in 1891 Merck & Co., Inc. is a global research-driven pharmaceutical company.
www.merck.com/mmhe/sec20.html

National Eye Institute
The National Eye Institute (NEI) was established by Congress in 1968 to protect and prolong the vision of the American people.
www.nei.nih.gov/health

UK

The Eyecare Trust
The Eyecare Trust is a registered charity that exists to raise awareness of all aspects of ocular health, the importance of regular eye care, and good eye wear.
Phone: 0845 129 5001
E-mail: info@eyecaretrust.org.uk
www.eyecaretrust.org.uk

EyeHelp
EyeHelp was formed to offer a reference point on eye problems and eye care. The features and articles are written by experts.
www.eyehelp.co.uk

Directgov
A Web site of the UK government for its citizens, providing information and services for the public.
www.direct.gov.uk/en/HealthAndWellBeing/HealthServices/ManagingYourHealthcare

CANADA

CNIB
Established in 1918, the Canadian National Institute for the Blind (CNIB) is the primary source of support and information for Canadians affected by vision loss.
Phone: (416) 486-2500
Toll-free (in Canada):
1-866-659-1843
www.cnib.ca

The Canadian Ophthalmological Society
The Canadian Ophthalmological Society (COS) was formed in 1937 and is recognized as the authority on eye care in Canada.
Phone: 613-729-6779
Fax: 613-729-7209
E-mail: cos@eyesite.ca
www.eyesite.ca

The Canadian Association of Optometrists
CAO is the professional association that represents Doctors of Optometry in Canada.
Phone: 613-235-7924
Toll Free (in Canada):
888-263-4676
Fax: 613-235-2025
www.opto.ca

The Canadian Orthoptic Society
The Canadian Orthoptic Society is a regulatory body consisting of ophthalmologists and orthoptists.
Fax: (306) 766-2769
E-mail: info@orthopticscanada.org
www.tcos.ca

The Foundation Fighting Blindness
A Canadian health charity that was founded in 1974 by a small group of families intent on finding a cure for the disease robbing their children of sight.
Phone: (416)360-4200
Fax: (416)360-0060
Toll-free (in Canada):
1-800-461-3331
E-mail: info@ffb.ca
www.ffb.ca

Canadian Guide Dogs for the Blind
Canadian Guide Dogs

for the Blind (CGDB) is a national, non-profit, registered, charitable organization that was founded in 1984.
Phone: (613) 692-7777
Fax: (613) 692-0650
E-mail: cgdb@sympatico.ca
www.guidedogs.ca

The Canadian Glaucoma Society

The Canadian Glaucoma Society offers a forum for Ophthalmologists with an interest in Glaucoma to exchange ideas.
www.eyesite.ca/cgs/

AUSTRALIA

HealthInsite

HealthInsite is an Australian Government initiative aimed at improving the health of Australians.
www.healthinsite.gov.au/topics/Eye_Health

Centre for Eye Research Australia (CERA)

CERA is affiliated with the Department of Ophthalmology at the University of Melbourne. It aims to improve the living conditions and lifestyles of people who are or may become vision-impaired.
http://cera.unimelb.edu.au

Glaucoma Australia

Glaucoma Australia aims to minimize visual disability from glaucoma. It offers counseling to sufferers, produces an informative newsletter, and holds regular support group meetings.
www.glaucoma.org.au

Macular Degeneration Foundation

A national organization based in Sydney whose key charter is to work for those with MD. Its programs are directed toward education, awareness, early detection and treatments, support services and representation.
Help Line: 1800 111 709
Phone: 02 9261 8900

Vision Australia

Vision Australia aims to improve the quality of life of people who are vision-impaired. It provides a diverse range of services tailored to a person's level of vision, most of them free of charge.
www.visionaustralia.org

NEW ZEALAND

Glaucoma NZ

Glaucoma NZ is a charitable trust that aims to eliminate blindness from glaucoma.
www.glaucoma.org.nz

Retina New Zealand

A self-help group that aims to promote public awareness of retinal degenerative disorders, to provide information and support, and to foster research leading to treatment and an eventual cure.
www.retina.org.nz

Royal New Zealand Foundation of the Blind

RNZFB is New Zealand's primary provider of vision-related habilitation and rehabilitation services to blind, deafblind, and vision-impaired people.
www.rnzfb.org.nz

SINGAPORE

Singapore National Eye Centre

SNEC commenced operations in 1990. It is the designated centre within the public sector healthcare network to co-ordinate the provision of specialised ophthalmological services.
www.snec.com.sg

National University Hospital Eye Surgery Centre

Established in 1986, the NUH Eye Surgery Centre has a team of eye surgeons offering a full array of diagnostic and therapeutic eye services.
www.nuheye.com

Singapore Eye Research Institute

The Singapore Eye Research Institute (SERI) is the national research institute for ophthalmic and vision research in Singapore.
www.seri.com.sg

Health Promotion Board

Established in 2001, the Health Promotion Board (HPB) has a vision to build a nation of healthy and happy people.
www.hpb.gov.sg/eyecare/default.aspx

Dept of Ophthalmology (Eye), Tan Tock Seng Hospital

TTSH's Department of Ophthalmology is the second largest unit in Singapore.
www.ttsh.com.sg/new/clinicalspecial/ophthalmology.php

MALAYSIA

The Tun Hussein Onn National Eye Hospital

THONEH is an eye hospital that was set up by YAB Tun Hussein Onn, who was the Chairman of Malaysian Association for the Blind (MAB).
www.thoneh.com

The Association of Malaysian Optometrists

Formed in 1984, the Association of Malaysian Optometrists is the profesional body that represents the primary eye care/optometry practice in Malaysia.
www.amoptom.org

National Eye Database

The National Eye Database (NED) is a service supported by the Ministry of Health (MOH) as an approach to collect health information.
www.acrm.org.my/ned/index.htm

PHILIPPINES

The American Eye Center

Established in 1995, the American Eye Center is an ophthalmic laser center for the treatment of nearsightedness, farsightedness, and astigmatism.
www.eyecenter.com.ph

Asian Eye Institute

Established in 2001, AEI provides a full range of specialized services.
www.asianeyeinstitute.com

EyeCare WeCare Foundation

The EyeCare WeCare Foundation is a registered, Christian charity that provides eye care services for free. The foundation targets the rural poor who do not have access to, or the financial resources for, vision services.
www.eyecarewecare.org

Index

Acknowledgments

Quantum would like to thank the following for the use of their pictures reproduced in this book:

Istock 2, 10, 21, 25, 31, 31, 36, 37, 103, 116, 117, 119, 119, 119, 122, 136, 150, 151, 158

SPL 11, 12, 13, 14, 15, 16, 19, 19, 19, 26, 28, 29, 32, 41, 46, 51, 53, 54, 55, 56, 59, 62, 64, 65, 67, 69, 71, 72, 75, 83, 91, 95, 96, 99, 101, 102, 105, 110, 125, 125, 125, 128, 129, 130, 131, 137, 140, 140, 141, 141, 142, 144, 144, 145, 146, 148, 149, 152, 154, 159, 162

Corbis 18, 23, 39, 100

Alamy 35, 38, 43, 47, 73, 74, 82, 113, 125, 134

NEI 50, 57, 61, 61, 84, 86, 86, 155

Fotosearch 107

Photolibrary 124, 133

All other photographs and illustrations are the copyright of Quantum. While every effort has been made to credit contributors, Quantum would like to apologize should there have been any omissions or errors – and would be pleased to make the appropriate correction for future editions of the book.